Does Your Lunch
Pack Punch?

A cookbook for the crunch & munch bunch

Does Your Lunch
Pack Punch?

A cookbook for the crunch & munch bunch

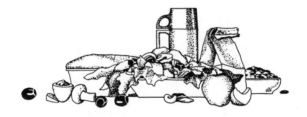

Robin Toth & Jacqueline Hostage

BETTERWAY PUBLICATIONS, INC.
White Hall, Virginia

First Printing: September, 1983

Published by Betterway Publications, Inc.
White Hall, VA 22987

Distributed to the book trade by
The Berkshire Traveller Press
Stockbridge, MA 01262

Cover design by Marion Reynolds
Typography by Typecasting

Library of Congress Cataloging in Publication Data

Toth, Robin
    Does your lunch pack punch for the crunch &
munch bunch?

    Includes index.
    1. Cookery (Natural foods)   2. Snack foods.
I. Hostage, Jacqueline E.   II. Title.
TX741.T67   1983   641.5   82-24512
ISBN 0-932620-20-5 (pbk.)

Printed in the United States of America

To all the big and little lunch munchers in our lives.

Contents

Introduction

If you're a brown bagger or thinking of becoming one...you're smart. That's what a recent market research survey tells us. You are better educated than people who don't brown bag ("better educated" doesn't always mean "smarter," but you are that, too; we'll tell you why in a minute). You also have more money and you are helping yourself maintain that status by not eating out as often.

One thing you are not, however, is exclusive. 80 million Americans regularly tote a home-prepared lunch. An estimated 34 million "brown bagged" lunches are eaten *every* work day. That's 9 billion lunches a year. Of course millions of kids take their lunches to school every day, too, but 70% of brown baggers are adults. And 40% of them are women. In fact—and this will be the last statistic—85% of America's working women carry their lunch.

We don't know—statistically—how many home-working women "brown bag" but more and more women are choosing to pack extra lunches in the morning for themselves and their preschoolers who are still at home. With lunch in the refrigerator or packed to travel, there is no need to rush back from the park or to miss an inspiring hour at one of the library or gallery lunchtime "brown bag" talks that are becoming so popular in so many areas.

It has always been easier to make choices at home—a chef's salad for lunch, for example, instead of a sandwich and chips—but now brown baggers can do that, too. A wonderful variety of packaging materials makes it possible for you to carry a good "home quality" lunch at prices no restaurant or cafeteria can match. It enables you to eat better and to allow for dietary considerations, if that is a current concern, by toting natural foods, fresh vegetables, salads, fruits, and home-baked whole-grain breads and desserts that are light on sugar.

And you get an added bonus. *You* choose where and how you spend your lunch hour; shopping...playing cards with friends...at the park ...or at a lunchtime lecture or musical program where lunch munchers are specifically invited. Just another way to benefit from the mobility and selectivity your carried meal provides.

This is a "home or away" lunch cookbook for everyone—brown baggers, homeworkers, and kids—who wants to eat nutritiously and well, and have a good time doing it. There are hundreds of terrific recipes, dozens of menu ideas, and some concise nutrition information in these pages—plus some really practical suggestions as to how you might organize your kitchen to make it a truly efficient lunch preparation center. The lunches you fix for yourself and your family can be better, more varied, cheaper, and a lot more fun. Please enjoy this book—and all the good lunches that follow—wherever you eat them.

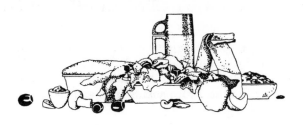

1: The Bag It, Box It, Tote It Guide

Home Take-Out Center Checklist
Guide to Containers for Packaging
Stocking up for Lunch-time: Pantry Checklist
Packaging Meals to Go
Take Out Food Safety Tips
Tips for the Budget-Conscious

Whether you prepare lunches to go the night before or in the morning, you can do it more easily if you have a work area dedicated to that function. A location close to the refrigerator is good; space between the refrigerator and the sink is even better. If you organize it efficiently, it need not be a very large area; two or three running feet of well-positioned counter space should be adequate.

Before you set up your lunch preparation area, go over the *Home Take-Out Center Checklist* on the next page. Once you know what you will need to make your lunch-fixing routine as pleasant and painless as possible, you'll have a pretty good idea what your counter space, drawer, and cabinet needs will be. Of course the number of brown baggers in your home will be a factor in your planning but—even if lunches-to-go are not a daily necessity—you will find a well-planned "take-out center" almost equally good as a packaging center for leftovers and foods to be frozen for planned-ahead meals.

Most of us enjoy fresh and natural foods. If these are to retain their freshness and appetizing appearance, you will want to package them "to go" with special care. Fortunately, the packaging industry has stayed abreast of our changing eating habits. A few dollars invested in containers of the right size, shape, and function will ensure that lunches travel in the style they require to retain their freshness and appeal.

HOME TAKE-OUT CENTER CHECKLIST

WRAPS
- [ ] **plastic wrap:** freezer or microwave safe wrap serves more uses
- [ ] **aluminum foil:** for sandwiches to be heated in conventional ovens
- [ ] **waxed paper:** for sandwiches to be heated in microwave ovens
- [ ] **sandwich bags:** use them for packing fruit and cookies, too

VACUUM CONTAINERS
- [ ] **thermos bottles:** choose standard neck bottles for carrying cold or hot liquids; wide-mouth for soups, stews, spaghetti, etc. Commonly available sizes include the ½ pint, pint, quart standard neck and the 10-ounce, pint, and quart wide mouth. Thermos cases are available in plastic, stainless steel, steel, or aluminum. Liners may be glass vacuum insulated (not recommended for children), non-breakable urethane insulated, or stainless steel.
- [ ] **thermos jars:** use jars for solid foods like salads, dips, finger foods, etc. Available in 6- and 10-ounce sizes.

PLASTIC FOOD CONTAINERS
- [ ] **2-ounce size:** perfect for salad dressing, relishes, dessert toppings
- [ ] **4–4½-ounce size:** for fruit, pudding, gelatin desserts, condiments, sauces, dips, sandwich fillings carried separately
- [ ] **6–8–12-ounce sizes:** side salads, "finger" salads
- [ ] **28–40-ounce size:** main dish salads

UTENSILS
- [ ] **sharp knives:** store these safely in a wooden knife rack or on a magnetic rack close to your preparation center
- [ ] **spreader** or **spatula:** for making quick work of sandwiches
- [ ] **bottle** or **can opener:** magnetized so it's readily available
- [ ] **cutting board:** select one you can sterilize easily

MISCELLANEOUS
- [ ] **refrigerants:** these handy, reusable "ice packs" now come in a lunch box size. They contain a gel that freezes solidly in your freezer; one can maintain the temperature in a lunch box for hours.
- [ ] **paper napkins:** add a supply of pre-moistened packaged "towelettes," too; they are especially good for after-lunch cleanups
- [ ] **plastic "silverware":** don't risk losing your stainless steel flatware; *everyone* forgets to bring the spoon home
- [ ] **paper towels:** for quick cleanups and disposable picnic "placemats"
- [ ] **salt and pepper:** packets or small containers (or "spepper"—just mix the two in the proportions you like)
- [ ] **lunch kits:** choose from rigid plastic, aluminum, or steel boxes, soft insulated totes, and rigid foam insulated coolers—or tuck a securely wrapped lunch in an over-sized purse, waterproof knapsack, or attaché case. And there is always the brown bag—plain or insulated.

GUIDE TO CONTAINERS AND MATERIALS

We have described and illustrated a sampling of the containers available to help you keep carried lunches fresher, tastier, and safer to eat. If you cannot find a particular product, write to the manufacturer for the name of the nearest dealer or distributor. You'll find that hardware stores and mail order catalogs often have the most extensive selections of lunch packing items.

Alabaster Prepare/Serve/Store Bowls and Trendee Commuter Cup
Alabaster Industries
P. O. Box 429
Alabaster, AL 35007

Alabaster's Prepare/Serve/Store bowls (but *not* their air tight covers) are safe for use in microwave ovens. These are available in a wide choice of sizes. Lunch toters will find the 10-, 16-, and 28-ounce rounds and the 16-ounce oblong the most useful. The Trendee Commuter Cup has a base that can be attached permanently to any smooth surface in your car, boat or camper to provide a non-spill holder for your hot beverage. A sipper lid allows you to drink without removing the lid. (*Commuter Cup not recommended for microwave use.*)

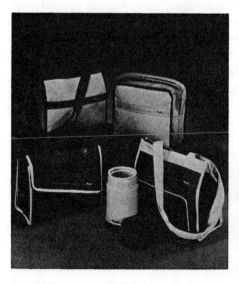

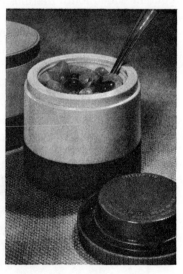

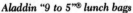

Aladdin "9 to 5"® lunch bags   *Aladdin Thermos Jar*

Aladdin Vacuum Bottles, Insulated Products, and Lunch Kits
Aladdin Industries, Inc.
Nashville, TN 37210

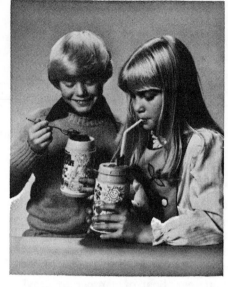

Aladdin vacuum bottles include standard neck and wide mouth bottles, in a wide range of sizes. Some features include Pump-a-Drink® tops and Tote 'n' Pour handles. Aladdin's Thermo Jar comes with a unique Freezer Lid top that is filled with pure, distilled water and permanently sealed; placing the lid in the freezer will freeze the water and enable the jar to keep any food refreshingly cold for hours. *None recommended for microwave use.*

Aladdin Pop-Top™ wide mouth thermos bottles

Lunch kits for children feature cartoon characters and contain wide-mouth thermos bottles—great for toting hot or cold solid foods that can be eaten right out of the bottle (some "wide-mouths" feature pop-up spouts that allow kids to drink right out of the bottle—with or without a straw). Lunch kits for men and women come in a variety of styles; the "9 to 5"® lunch bags for women (featuring zipper or Velcro® closures and carrying straps) are real winners.

Freezette® Storage Containers, Micro-ette® Micro-Mugs
Republic Molding Corporation
Chicago, IL 60648

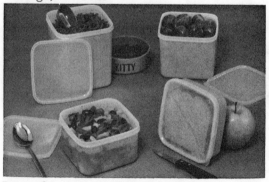

Freezette® containers with Snap-Lok covers

Freezette® plastic containers come in a wide variety of styles and sizes for the lunch toter, including sandwich containers, pie-wedge containers, Snap-Lok containers that are ideal for salads, and Twist-Top jars and beverage bottles in sizes from 8

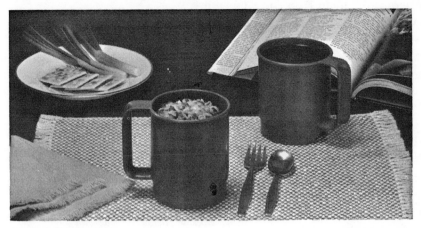
Micro-ette® Micro-Mugs

ounces to 1 gallon. *Not recommended for microwave use.*

Micro-ette® Micro-Mugs are made in a generous 20-ounce size that is ideal for beverages, soups (a mug will hold a regular can of soup, diluted to the extent most soup users prefer), and for cooking or reheating meals-in-a-mug. Dishwasher safe with a stay-cool handle for microwave use.

Hefty Microwave Food Containers
Mobil Chemical Company
Plastics Division
Macedon, NY 14502

Containers with clear thermo-plastic snap seal lids that store, stack, freeze, and are microwave and dishwasher safe. 1- and 1½-pint, 1- and 1½-quart sizes are handy for the lunch box.

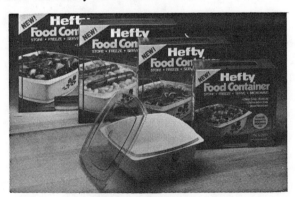
Hefty Food Containers

Microware® Main Dish and Side Dish
Anchor Hocking
Lancaster, OH 43130

Ideal for leftovers or main dishes that you want to reheat—at home or away. The 16-ounce Main Dish and 8-ounce Side Dish go—safely and attractively—from freezer to microwave oven to table. Their clear plastic lids make them great for toting snacks or tidbits too.

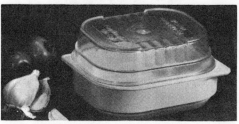

Anchor Hocking Microware® Side Dish

Rubbermaid® Plastic Containers and Microwave Cookware
Rubbermaid Industries
1147 Akron Road
Wooster, OH 44691

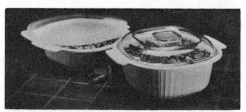

Rubbermaid® Microwave Cookware

Rubbermaid® Servin' Savers are sturdy 2-cup covered plastic containers—just the right size for freezing, storing, stacking, or toting sandwiches, side dishes, and tidbits. *Not recommended for microwave use.* The Rubbermaid line of Microwave Cookware contains a broad range of shapes and sizes but the lunch toter who wants to be able to utilize a microwave oven at her/his office or plant will find the most use for the 1- and 2-quart casseroles that offer both cooking lids *and* flexible storage lids.

Thermos® Vacuum Bottles, Insulated Products, and Lunch Kits
Thermos
Thermos Avenue
Norwich, CT 06360

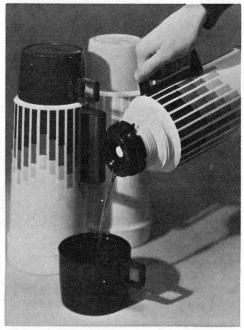

Thermos® vacuum bottle

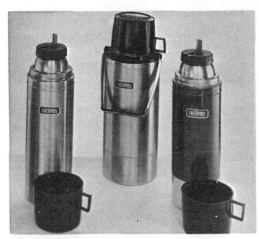

Stainless steel Thermos® vacuum bottles with
Flip 'n' Pour™ stoppers

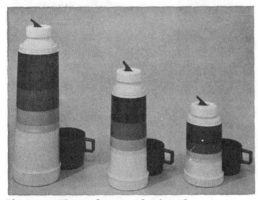

Plastic case Thermos® vacuum bottle with
Flip 'n' Pour™ stoppers

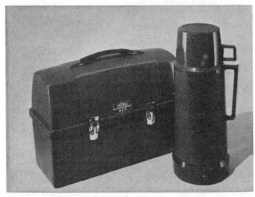

Thermos® Workman's Lunch Kit

Thermos® vacuum bottles and insulated products include ½ pint to 2-quart standard neck bottles and 10-ounce to 1-quart wide mouth jars. Bottle casings include plastic, steel, or aluminum and a choice of glass lined or unbreakable stainless steel linings. Features include Flip 'n' Pour™ stoppers, and Touch Top™ dispensers. Other insulated products include unbreakable Roughneck™ bottles designed for little hands; Snak Jars™ that are ideal for soups, fruits, salads, and desserts; spill-proof, insulated 10-ounce Go-Cups™. *None recommended for microwave use.*

Lunch kits for children feature cartoon characters and unbreakable bottles; kits for adults and older children are available in rigid plastic or insulated plastic or soft Fiberglas® insulated carrying cases.

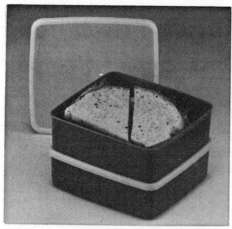

Tupperware Square-a-Way® Set

Tupperware
Tupperware Home Parties
Customer Relations
Department
P. O. Box 2353
Orlando, FL 32802

Wide variety of plastic containers for storing, freezing, serving and toting. Includes: Square-a-Way® containers for large sandwiches and finger foods; Seal-N-Serve® bowls in 2¼ cup and 3¼ cup capacities for salads and side dishes; Packette® divided containers (perfect for finger foods and dip), 2-ounce Midgets that are ideal for salad dressings and condiments; Tumbler Sets and Seals in 6, 8, 12, and 18-ounce sizes; 4½-ounce Snack Cups. *Not recommended for microwave use.*

Carrying kits include regular (for older children and adults) and mini (for younger children) Pak-N-Carry® Kits.

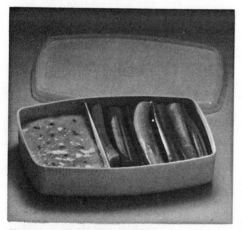

Tupperware Packette™ container

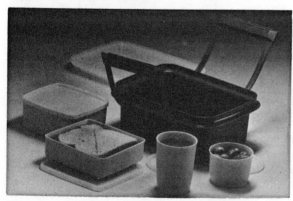

Tupperware Pack-N-Carry™ Kit

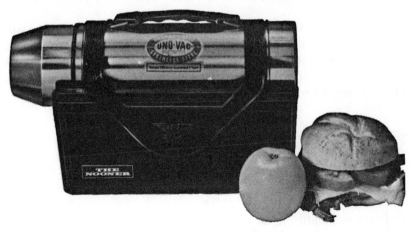

Uno-Vac® Nooner Combo

Uno-Vac® Vacuum Bottles, Wide Mouth Food Jars, and Lunch Kits
Union Manufacturing Co.
290 Pratt Street
Meriden, CT 06450

Uno-Vac® vacuum bottles and jars feature stainless steel linings and casings with plastic lined stainless steel cups and are warranteed for thermal efficiency for five years. *Not recomended for microwave use.*

   Lunch kits and insulated tote bags are well designed—primarily for the workman, sportsman, or older child.

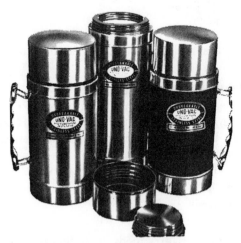

Uno-Vac® wide mouth thermal food jars

STOCKING UP FOR LUNCH-TIME: PANTRY CHECKLIST

Your "take out" kitchen can serve the variety of a cafeteria or health food restaurant—if you plan ahead. Stock your food storage areas with easily prepared luncheon foods to eliminate early morning hassles as well as the temptation to opt for an over-priced coffee shop meal. Here are some suggestions to broaden your take-out menu.

PANTRY*

☐ Basic staples: whole-grain or enriched unbleached flours, baking powder, baking soda, flavoring extracts, cocoa or carob, plain gelatin, herbs, spices, yeast, oil, vinegar, condiments, relishes, and pickles
☐ Beans and lentils, dried
☐ Bulgur (cracked wheat) or Kasha (buckwheat groats)
☐ Cereals, preferably rolled oats, rye or other steel cut varieties
☐ Crackers and cookies, preferably homemade
☐ Fruit, natural, unsweetened, canned and dried
☐ Grains and seeds for sprouting
☐ Honey, maple syrup, or unsulfured molasses for sweetening
☐ Juices, vegetable and unsweetened fruit, small cans or boxes
☐ Mayonnaise and salad dressings
☐ Nuts and seeds, preferably unsalted
☐ Peanut butter, natural, *not* hydrogenated
☐ Puddings, 5-ounce individual serving size
☐ Rice, brown or natural
☐ Soups, single serving sizes
☐ Tamari or soy sauce
☐ Tuna, water pack; other canned fish or seafood
☐ Vegetables, beans, and chick peas, canned, for quick salads or main dishes

REFRIGERATOR OR FREEZER

☐ Basic staples: eggs, poultry, fish, meats, butter or margarine
☐ Cheeses, preferably *not* "processed" or "processed cheese food"
☐ Fruits, apples, bananas, oranges, and varieties in season
☐ Juices, unsweetened
☐ Sandwiches and sandwich fillings, soups, stews, etc., frozen
☐ Tofu and/or tempeh
☐ Vegetables, fresh and frozen
☐ Yogurt, plain

*Remember that many pantry foods, including peanut butter, should be stored in the refrigerator after opening.

PACKAGING MEALS TO GO

ASSEMBLY LINE SANDWICHES

Start with softened butter or margarine (or one of the seasoned butters on page 46) and well chilled sandwich fillings.
Line up bread slices in rows, so that slices match in size.
Butter all slices right to the very edges to prevent filling from soaking into bread.
Place filling on slices in one row, spread to edges, close with matching slice of bread.
Cut sandwiches in halves or quarters; transfer to sandwich bags or center of a square of plastic wrap, foil, or waxed paper. Close bag tightly or wrap with drug store wrap. (That's the one where you bring the two long sides of the wrap together over the center of the sandwich and then fold the edges over and over until the fold rests against the sandwich. Fold leftover end corners toward each other and then tuck under.)
Refrigerate prepared sandwiches until time to pack in lunch box; keep perishable (especially meat, fish, poultry, or eggs) sandwiches cold until lunch time by adding a refrigerant or a can of frozen juice to the lunch box (juice will thaw in time for lunch).
Freeze the extra sandwiches you have made for future lunches.

Sandwich Tips:

Adults or older children may prefer to tote sandwich fillings separately (packaged in a prechilled thermos jar) for assembling at lunch time. This is particularly nice for fillings that might make the bread soggy.

Several thin slices of meat will make a more flavorful sandwich than one thick slice.

If you use your own homemade bread, store it (well wrapped) in the refrigerator for easier slicing.

FRESH FROM THE FREEZER LUNCHES

Prepare extra soup, chili, and stew when you cook. They are easily frozen in portion size containers for last minute heating before pouring into a vacuum bottle. Freeze leftover cooked meats or other "fillers" in sandwich size portions, all ready to slap between two slices of fresh buttered bread; for example, bread shaped packages of ham and cheese, chicken and crisp bacon slices, leftover cooked meats or meat/chicken/vegetable loaves. This trick eliminates the major objection to frozen sandwiches: the "off" flavor that bread develops so quickly in freezing.
Avoid using ingredients in sandwiches that could soak into bread or

change in texture or flavor: salad dressing, mayonnaise, jelly, egg whites, sour cream, cottage cheese, cream cheese, fresh raw vegetables. Substitute butter or margarine, mustard, catsup, relish, or chili sauce as a spread for the bread.

Package in materials that are suitable for freezing. If you plan to thaw or reheat in a microwave oven, make sure the packaging material or container is suitable for that as well. Freezer to oven to table containers are time savers.

Label sandwiches or containers with kind and date. A convenient way to freeze soups and stews is to use flat plastic sandwich boxes. When solidly frozen, pop out of the box, and wrap in freezer wrap. The packages will stack neatly in your freezer and the boxes will be ready for reuse. For easy access, stack in a separate container or wire freezer basket.

Plan to use frozen sandwiches within 2–3 weeks for best flavor. Soups, stews and other prepared foods taste best if used within 2–3 months.

Allow 2–3 hours for wrapped, frozen sandwiches to thaw at room temperature, 5–6 hours to thaw in the refrigerator. Most single serving size containers of food will thaw and reheat quickly in a microwave oven or over low heat.

Remember to add raw vegetables that lose their crispness—lettuce, tomatoes, celery, etc—just before eating.

SALADS THAT KEEP THEIR SNAP

Tossed green salads can be prepared ahead of time and retain their crispness. Other ingredients—meats, cheese, hardcooked eggs, tomatoes, salad dressing, etc.—can be used if they are packaged and carried separately for adding at the last minute. Start with well cleaned and drained salad greens and pile lightly into a large, single serving size covered container. Fold a white paper towel twice, place atop the salad greens, and cover tightly. Place container upside down in the refrigerator. (The towel will catch the last of the excess water from the greens and the humidity in the towel will keep the greens crisp!) When ready to tote, remove paper towel. For guaranteed crispness (and extra nutrients at lunch time), stash a container of frozen juice or yogurt amidst the greens and carry everything in an insulated lunch kit.

Molded salads carry well in small insulated thermos jars. There is no need to prechill the jars if you use the "quick-set" method of adding ice cubes and stirring until the gelatin begins to thicken. Stir in the remaining ingredients and pour into thermos jars. Seal. Refrigerate 1 hour or overnight.

TAKE OUT FOOD SAFETY TIPS

• Prevent food contamination and possible food poisoning by handling foods properly. Insist on strict cleanliness for anyone handling or preparing foods, as well as making sure that all utensils, containers, and work surfaces are clean. (A solution of 3 tablespoons liquid bleach in a quart of warm water will help to destroy bacteria on countertops and other surfaces.)

• Select and prepare foods for toted lunches carefully. Raw fruits and vegetables should be washed thoroughly. Foods should be prepared with the same fresh ingredients that you would choose for regular family meals and should be stored just as carefully. Hot dishes should be heated through completely before pouring into a preheated vacuum bottle or jar.

• Wash the tops of canned foods before opening or packing them in the lunch kit. (Cans may be covered with the residue of a pesticide or cleaning spray used in the store.)

• For safety's sake, don't recycle plastic wrap, foil, waxed paper, etc. Make sure that any recycled containers (baby food jars, plastic containers) used for carrying food are scrupulously clean and odor free.

• Keep vacuum bottles immaculate. Follow the directions for cleaning that came with your brand of vacuum bottles or jars or sanitize by half filling with soapy water and scrubbing with a soft bottle brush. Fill with boiling water, cover, and let stand a few minutes before pouring out and rinsing well. Between uses, rinse, dry, and store with cup and stopper removed. Never wash in an automatic dishwasher.

• Before filling a vacuum container with a hot or cold beverage or food, heat the inside with boiling water or chill it with ice water (or by placing open bottle in refrigerator for 15 minutes); food will retain its desired temperature longer.

• Prepare cold foods long enough ahead so that they will be well chilled before packing in the thermos or other container. Heat hot foods thoroughly before pouring into preheated thermos.

• Keep perishable cold foods cold (40°), and perishable hot foods, hot. We like to test our vacuum containers occasionally for efficiency by using an instant thermometer to check the temperature of food (or use boiling water) in the thermos after it has stood for several hours. When a thermos loses its ability to retain temperatures, it may just need a replacement stopper or cap.

• Remind family members of the importance of caring for their lunches. That means, refrigerating cold lunches, if facilities are available, and *not* leaving their lunch kits on a sunny windowsill or on the back seat of the car on a hot day. (And, if you are *really* lucky, they'll rinse out their thermos bottles after lunch!)

• Foods retain their temperature better when they fill the thermos completely. If your food doesn't fill the thermos, lay a piece of aluminum foil on top of the food: the extra insulation will keep it hotter, longer.

• Check any precautions that were included with your brand of vacuum bottle: glass lined bottles, for example, are not recommended for children; some manufacturers recommend you not eat directly from their vacuum bottles.

• Carbonated beverages are not recommended for vacuum bottles; the pressure created by the gases used for carbonation can cause leakage.

TIPS FOR THE BUDGET CONSCIOUS

• Get together with your co-workers and plan an occasional day where each person brings enough of one food item to serve everyone. Lunch for the bunch can be a money saver as well as fun. Or, take turns sharing a lunch with another friend.

• Marinate leftover cooked vegetables from dinner in a vinaigrette or Italian dressing. Refrigerate for a tasty luncheon salad the next day.

• Don't discard that jar of leftover pickle juice. Add sliced julienne cut carrots and let stand at least a day.

• Save the insulated bags in which the supermarket packages your ice-cream. One can give your lunch added protection on a hot day.

• Clean, empty pill bottles are good for travelling salt, no-salt seasoning, pepper, sugar substitutes, etc.

• Picnics are fun—until it's time to pack up and go home. Create a disposable picnic cooler by freezing water filled coffee cans. Then place one large paper bag inside another and insulate your "cooler" by slipping several thicknesses of newspaper *between* the two bags. Line the whole thing with a plastic bag; place several cans of ice in the bottom and put your food (packaged in disposable containers, of course!)— tucking small or perishable items between the coffee cans. After your picnic, just pile the waste in the plastic bag—ice cans included—and drop it in the nearest trash barrel.

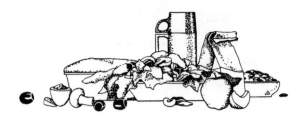

2: Breakfast at Home...
on the Run...at Work

Fruits
Cereals-to-Go
Quiches and other Egg Dishes
Breakfast Puddings
Quick Breads and Muffins
Breakfast Cookies and Take-a-Shakes

Breakfast ideas in a lunch cookbook for brown baggers? Of course! If you're the type who can't stand the sight of food first thing in the morning or have kids who rush off insisting they haven't time for breakfast, pack a nutritious mid-morning snack.

The nighttime "fast" leaves blood sugar (glucose) levels at a low point. Studies show that children and adults who skip breakfast show a poorer attitude toward work and become less efficient as the morning progresses. So, if you or those you love are not getting 25% of the day's total calories at breakfast-time, bag it and take it or send it!

Make morning mealtime fun again. Man's breakfast eating habits have come a long way since the early Middle Ages when breakfast consisted merely of bread and ale. Few of us have the appetite for the formidable old English groaning board of kippers, finnan haddie, kedgeree, roast beef, kidneys, and a variety of cakes and other English breakfast staples. But breakfast doesn't have to be the traditional American breakfast of juice and cereal or bacon and eggs either. Consider: a mug of hot potato or tomato soup, Brown Rice Custard topped with fresh fruit, a light cream cheese sandwich on date and nut bread, fruit and nut turnovers that are light on sugar and high on nutrition, or a nutrition packed Breakfast Cookie and a frothy milk or fruit shake.

[25]

Morning Fruit Cup

Unsweetened pineapple tid-bits can form the base for fruit cup using any of your favorite fruits that are in season.

> 1 8-ounce can unsweetened pineapple tid-bits
> 1 cup fresh orange sections
> 1 medium apple, unpeeled, diced
> ½ cup seedless grapes

Combine fruits gently. Chill several hours or overnight. (Make sure apple is completely covered with liquid to prevent darkening.) Makes 4 servings.

Package individual servings in 6-ounce thermos jars.

Grapefruit Surprise

The "surprise" is in the delicious flavor of this unusual combination of fruits.

> 2 grapefruit
> 1 cup sliced strawberries
> 2 tablespoons sugar or honey

Wash and halve grapefruit; remove sections. Place in bowl with 1 tablespoon of the sugar or honey; cover and refrigerate. Remove inner membrane from grapefruit shells and reserve shells (store in refrigerator).

Combine strawberries with remaining 1 tablespoon sugar or honey. Chill several hours or overnight.

To serve, fill reserved shells with grapefruit and spoon strawberries over.

Old-fashioned Prunes

So old-fashioned that it's new again...and still good!

> 1 1-pound box whole, pitted prunes
> 1½ cups apple juice
> 2 tablespoons lemon juice
> 2 tablespoons honey

Bring all ingredients to a boil and simmer, covered, 5 minutes. Pour into a covered jar or bowl and refrigerate until needed. Good warm, too.

Package in small insulated thermos jar. For reheating before serving, carry in microwave safe covered container.

Fall Fruit Compote

Not only good for breakfast over cooked cereal, but also for lunch over cooked grains, or as a dessert or nutritious snack.

> *3-4 apples, preferably tart*
> *3 pears*
> *2 oranges*
> *⅓ cup raisins*
> *⅓ cup coarsely chopped almonds*
> *¾ cup maple syrup*
> *1 teaspoon almond extract*
> *2 tablespoons water or orange juice*

Preheat oven to 350°. Wash, core, and peel apples and pears. Peel oranges, remove seeds, and chop coarsely. Combine all ingredients in a lightly greased baking dish. Cover and bake 45–50 minutes. Serve warm or cold.

Breakfast Quiche-to-go

Fast and fabulous.

> *pastry for 9-inch pie shell*
> *1½ cups plain yogurt*
> *1 tablespoon prepared horseradish*
> *4 eggs*
> *½ teaspoon Worcestershire sauce*
> *1 teaspoon salt or tamari sauce*
> *1 cup grated Swiss, Cheddar, or other firm cheese*
> *1 cup chopped scallions*

Preheat oven to 375°. Line an 8-inch square baking pan with the pastry. Mix all remaining ingredients with a whisk or wooden spoon. Pour into pastry lined pan. Bake 30 to 45 minutes. Cut into squares. Good hot, warm, or cold.

Vary the flavor of this recipe by substituting 1 tablespoon of Cognac or Sherry and ½ teaspoon rosemary for the prepared horseradish. Stir in ½ cup cherry tomato halves, if desired.

To save time in the morning prepare the pie shell and mix the filling ingredients the night before. Store in refrigerator. In the morning, just pour the filling into the prepared baking pan and bake while you are getting ready for work.

All-In-One Microwave Breakfast

This can be prepared the night before and refrigerated until ready to bake and serve.

> 1 egg
> ½ cup milk
> ⅛ teaspoon salt
> ¼ teaspoon dry mustard
> 1 cup soft bread cubes (½-inch cubes)
> ¼ cup diced cooked ham
> 2 tablespoons grated Cheddar or Monterey Jack cheese

In mixing bowl beat eggs slightly. Blend in milk, mustard, salt. Stir in bread and ham. Pour into microwave safe mug or 5–6-inch bowl. Sprinkle with cheese. Cover with plastic wrap, piercing the wrap in several places to allow steam to escape. Microwave at Medium for 6–7 minutes, or until center is set. Let stand for 1 minute.

Tote only if you can keep this well chilled and plan to bake within the hour.

Western Style Breakfast Pizza

This is a real winner—worth the short time it takes to prepare.

> 1 8-ounce can refrigerated crescent roll dough
> 2 tablespoons mayonnaise
> 1 teaspoon prepared mustard
> 1 teaspoon oil
> ¼ pound bacon, cooked, drained, and crumbled
> ¼ cup finely chopped onion
> ¼ cup finely chopped green pepper
> 1 cup sliced fresh mushrooms
> 4 eggs
> ¼ cup water
> Salt and pepper to taste

Preheat oven to 400°. Spread dough over bottom of 11–12-inch pizza pan, patting edges together to form a crust and building up edges to form a rim. Combine mayonnaise, mustard, and oil; spread on crust. Sprinkle crust with bacon and vegetables. Beat eggs, salt, pepper, and water together; pour over top of pizza. Bake 25 minutes or until puffed and browned.

Busy Day Tip: Beat the morning rush by substituting ½ cup diced cooked ham or by cooking the bacon the night before.

Crusted Oven Omelet

Here's an omelet you can even eat on your way out the door.

10-inch pastry shell (prebaked for 5 minutes in a 400° oven and
  cooled.)
1 cup water
1 cup chicken or vegetable broth
½ cup flour
¼ cup soft margarine
1 cup grated cheese (Swiss or Monterey Jack is good)
5 eggs, slightly beaten
¼ teaspoon salt
¼ teaspoon dry mustard
¼ teaspoon freshly grated black pepper

Preheat oven to 400°. In small saucepan, carefully stir liquids into flour
until smooth. Bring to a boil and cook and stir until thick. Remove
from heat. Add margarine and stir until blended. Add all remaining
ingredients; pour into pie shell. Bake 30 minutes. Cut into 6–8 wedges.

All-Purpose Granola

This recipe is particularly good for just "munching."

4 cups oatmeal
½ cup wheat germ
1 cup sunflower seeds
¾ cup chopped nuts
¾ cup raisins and/or chopped dates
½ cup corn oil
½ cup honey or brown sugar
2 teaspoons vanilla

Preheat oven to 225°. Combine oatmeal and wheat germ in large bowl.
Mix together oil, honey or brown sugar, and vanilla. Drizzle over
cereals and mix well; spread on oiled baking sheet. Bake 45 minutes.
Stir in remaining ingredients; bake 15 minutes longer. Cool before storing in covered jar or plastic bags.

Vary to suit your own tastes by changing ingredients or proportions.
Other nuts or dried fruits can be used: bran, rolled rye or whole-wheat,
sesame seeds, coconut, or almost any grain, seed, nut, or dried fruit that
you have on hand.

Apple Granola

Low on sweeteners—high on flavor.

3 cups oatmeal
½ cup coconut
½ cup sunflower seeds
1 cup chopped walnuts
1 teaspoon cinnamon
⅔ cup oil
1 6-ounce can apple juice concentrate, thawed
¼ cup honey (optional)
1 cup chopped dried apples

Preheat oven to 300°. Combine all ingredients, *except* apples, and place on greased cookie sheet or baking pan. Bake 15 minutes. Stir in apples; bake 15–20 minutes longer. Cool before storing in covered jar or plastic bags.

Hot 'n' Spicy Apple Granola

A nice change for winter mornings.

1 cup Apple Granola
1 cup apple juice
1 tablespoon butter
1 tablespoon brown sugar or maple syrup
⅛ teaspoon cinnamon

Combine all ingredients in heavy saucepan. Bring to a boil over medium heat; reduce heat and simmer 1 minute, stirring frequently. Serve with soy or dairy milk, if desired.

Breakfast-to-Go

This "winter" breakfast tastes light and fresh enough for summer. Add a spoonful of sweetener with the boiling water, if desired.

½ cup oatmeal
½ cup minced apple
2 tablespoons sunflower seeds
½ teaspoon allspice
1 cup boiling water

Combine ingredients and pour into thermos bottle. Cap tightly. Let stand overnight.

"Cold" Cereal

Similar to the Swiss "muesli," this cereal needs only the addition of a bit of milk or fruit juice to make it a treat. It has a fresh flavor that you can't get out of a package.

¼ cup rolled rye
3 tablespoons raisins
2 tablespoons chopped almonds
4 tablespoons shredded or flaked coconut
4 tablespoons water
1 small unpeeled apple, chopped

Combine all ingredients, *except* apple. Refrigerate, covered, overnight. When ready to serve or package for toting, stir in chopped apple. Makes 2 servings.

Package desired amount in small insulated thermos jar.

Vary by substituting oat or wheat flakes, wheat germ, walnuts or pecans. Try diced mixed dried fruit, dates, or prunes instead of raisins; fresh pear instead of apple.

Breakfast Bulgur

Make this in the thermos the night before for a grab-it-and-run breakfast the next morning.

¼ cup bulgur
¼ teaspoon salt
1 tablespoon honey
¼ teaspoon vanilla
2 tablespoons chopped dried apples or raisins
1 tablespoon chopped walnuts
¾ cup boiling apple juice or water

Combine all ingredients, *except* apple juice or water, in a preheated 10-ounce wide-mouth thermos. Pour in rapidly boiling water; cover tightly and shake well. Turn on its side and let stand overnight. Add milk at serving time, if desired, but it really isn't needed.

Multiple servings can be cooked on top of the stove by doubling and combining all ingredients in a saucepan. Boil 5 minutes; cover, simmer 15 minutes. Let stand, covered, for an additional 10 minutes before serving.

Old-fashioned Brown Rice Custard

Here is another way to use up leftover rice. Natural brown rice and cereal with wholesome honey add up to a nutritious breakfast (or dessert).

½ cup uncooked natural brown rice
1 cup natural cereal with raisins and dates
2 cups milk, scalded
2 eggs, lightly beaten
⅓ cup honey or maple syrup
2 tablespoons butter or margarine
1 teaspoon vanilla
½ teaspoon salt
½ teaspoon ground nutmeg

Cook the brown rice according to package directions using ½ teaspoon salt. Or, use 1½ cups cooked brown rice.

Preheat oven to 350°. Pour the cereal into a 1½-quart casserole. Add the cooked rice to the scalded milk. Stir in the eggs, honey, butter or margarine, vanilla, salt, and nutmeg. Pour mixture over cereal. Place casserole into shallow pan and pour hot water to 1-inch from the top of the casserole. Bake, uncovered, for 30 minutes. Stir gently and bake another 20 minutes or until knife inserted near the center comes out clean. Makes about 8 servings.

Busy Day Variation: Combine in a heavy saucepan 1 cup cooked rice, 1 cup milk, 2 tablespoons nonfat dry milk, 2 tablespoons brown sugar, 1 teaspoon vanilla, and a dash of nutmeg. Cook and stir over medium heat for about 5 minutes or until mixture is thick and creamy. Serve warm or cold with fruit, if desired.

Foxy Quick Brown Rice Tip: Presoaking your brown rice can cut cooking time from 1 hour to 20 minutes. Just stir the rice into 2½ cups water for *each* cup of rice used. Let stand at least 2 hours at room temperature (or refrigerate for 6–24 hours). When ready to cook, bring rice and water to a boil, cover pan, and simmer 17–20 minutes or until all water is absorbed.

Overnight Bread Pudding

Prepare this the night before and bake it in the morning to serve warm or bake it the night before and chill in the refrigerator overnight.

    4-5 slices (day old or stale) raisin bread
    2 tablespoons soft butter or margarine
    ¼ cup raisins
    3 eggs, well beaten
    3 cups milk
    ⅓ cup brown sugar
    ⅛ teaspoon salt
    ¼ teaspoon ground nutmeg
    2 teaspoons vanilla

Spread the slices of bread with butter or margarine. Stack the buttered slices and cut into 1-1½ inch squares; scatter in greased 8 × 8 × 2 baking dish. Sprinkle with raisins. Combine remaining ingredients; pour over bread. Cover tightly with plastic wrap. Let stand 1-12 hours in refrigerator.

Preheat oven to 350°. Bake 40 minutes or until puffed and browned and knife inserted in pudding comes out clean. Cool 10-15 minutes or chill in refrigerator before serving.

Heavenly Noodle Kugel

Make this the night before and pop it into the oven as soon as you get up. Good warm or cold, with or without milk poured over.

    6 ounces wide noodles
    1 cup yogurt or sour cream
    1 cup cottage cheese
    2 eggs, well beaten
    ½ cup brown sugar
    4 tablespoons melted butter or margarine
    1 15-ounce can crushed pineapple, undrained
    ¼ cup chopped nuts (optional)
    ¼ teaspoon cinnamon

Cook noodles according to package directions; rinse with cold water and drain well. Combine noodles with remaining ingredients and place in a greased shallow 2-quart baking dish. Refrigerate for several hours or overnight if not baking immediately.

Preheat oven to 375°. Bake 1 hour, 15 minutes.

Cornbread

Add crunch. Sprinkle sesame or sunflower seeds on top before baking.

1 cup wholewheat flour
¾ cup cornmeal
1 tablespoon baking powder
½ teaspoon salt
¼ cup maple syrup or honey
½ cup water or milk
⅓ cup oil, preferably corn oil
1 egg

Preheat oven to 425°. Combine dry ingredients in mixing bowl. Add remaining ingredients; stir just until blended (batter will be lumpy). Spoon into greased 8 × 8 × 2-inch pan. Bake 25–30 minutes. Cool slightly in pan; cut into squares to serve.

Variation: To make handy cakes for your toaster, cut cornbread into 6 pieces; split each piece in half. Cool completely before wrapping individually and freezing. No need to thaw before toasting or reheating in microwave oven.

Banana Muffins

Easier to tote than banana bread, these are equally tempting. Be sure to use very ripe bananas for the best flavor.

1 cup unbleached all-purpose flour
¼ cup sugar
2½ teaspoons baking powder
½ teaspoon baking soda
½ teaspoon salt
½ teaspoon cinnamon
¼ teaspoon nutmeg
½ cup oatmeal
1 cup mashed banana
½ cup milk
¼ cup oil or melted margarine
1 egg, beaten
½ cup chopped nuts (optional)

Preheat oven to 425°. Combine dry ingredients in large bowl. Blend in blender or stir together remaining ingredients. Add to dry ingredients, stirring just until moistened. Fill greased and floured medium-size muffin pans using about ¼ cup batter in each cup. Bake 15 minutes or until done. Makes 12 muffins.

Blueberry Wheat Muffins

We bet this will become a favorite in your home, too!

1 ½ cups whole-wheat flour
2 teaspoons baking powder
½ teaspoon salt
¼ cup plain wheat germ
1 egg
½ cup milk
¼ cup honey
¼ cup margarine, melted and cooled
1 cup blueberries

Preheat oven to 400°. Sift together flour, baking powder, and salt. Stir in wheat germ. In separate bowl, beat egg until thick. Add milk and honey; beat well. Stir in margarine.

Add liquid ingredients to dry ingredients; stir until moistened. Fold in blueberries. Turn into medium-size paper-lined muffin pans, filling ⅔ full. Bake 20–25 minutes or until done. Makes 12.

Orange Muffins

Perfect with scrambled eggs, these are scrumptious enough for dessert as well.

2 tablespoons each: brown sugar
                       grated coconut
                       finely chopped nuts
½ teaspoon grated orange rind
¼ teaspoon allspice
2 eggs, lightly beaten
¼ cup brown sugar
¼ cup oil
⅔ cup orange juice, preferably fresh
1 tablespoon grated orange rind
2 cups unbleached all-purpose flour
2 teaspoons baking powder
½ teaspoon salt

Preheat oven to 400°. Mix together first five ingredients for topping and set aside. Combine eggs, sugar, oil, orange juice, and orange rind in a medium bowl; stir to blend. Sift dry ingredients onto egg mixture; blend gently just until all ingredients are moistened. Spoon into 12 paper-lined medium-size muffin pans. Sprinkle with topping. Bake 15 minutes. Turn out onto wire rack to cool.

Bran Orange Muffins

These are lighter and more delicate than bran muffins usually are.

⅔ cup orange juice
1½ teaspoons grated orange rind
1 egg
2 tablespoons oil
1 cup bran cereal
⅔ cup unbleached all-purpose flour
1½ teaspoons baking powder
¼ teaspoon salt
¼ cup sugar
¼ cup chopped nuts (optional)

Preheat oven to 400°. Beat together first four ingredients; stir in bran cereal. Let stand 5 minutes. Combine remaining ingredients; add to bran mixture, stirring just until dry ingredients are moistened. Turn into medium-size paper-lined muffin tins, filling ⅔ full. Bake 12–15 minutes or until done. Makes 12.

Apple Butter Muffins

Fun to eat and lower in calories than most muffins.

1¾ cups wholewheat flour
1 tablespoon baking powder
¼ teaspoon salt
½ teaspoon lemon or vanilla extract
2 tablespoons maple syrup
⅓ cup oil
¾ cup apple juice or milk
⅓ cup apple butter (about)

Preheat oven to 400°. Combine dry ingredients in large bowl. Mix together remaining ingredients, *except apple butter.* Make a well in the middle of the dry ingredients and add combined remaining ingredients; mix just until blended. Using two-thirds of the batter, partially fill 12 greased muffin cups. Spoon 1 heaping teaspoon of apple butter on top of each muffin; cover with remaining batter. Bake about 18–20 minutes.

Raisin and Bran Muffins

A nutritious version of an old favorite.

> 2 cups Nutri-Grain Raisin Bran
> 1 ½ cups whole-wheat flour
> ¼ teaspoon salt
> 1 teaspoon allspice
> 1 ¼ teaspoons baking soda
> ½ cup maple syrup
> ½ cup crumbled tofu or cottage cheese
> ½ cup plain yogurt
> ¼ cup oil
> ¼ cup raisins or currants
> ¼ cup chopped nuts

Preheat oven to 375°. Place yogurt, tofu or cottage cheese, oil, and maple syrup in blender; blend just until smooth. Combine dry ingredients in large bowl. Pour over the blended ingredients and mix gently. Fold in raisins or currants and nuts. Spoon into 12 large or 36 small well-oiled muffin tins. Bake 15–20 minutes.

Oatmeal Muffins

These are so light that you won't miss the egg. (Good news for cholesterol watchers.)

> 1 cup rolled oats
> ¼ cup plain yogurt
> ¾ cup warm water
> ½ cup oil
> 1 cup whole-wheat flour
> 1 tablespoon baking powder
> ½ teaspoon baking soda
> 1 tablespoon grated orange or lemon rind
> 1 teaspoon orange or lemon extract
> ¼ cup honey
> ¼ cup sunflower seeds

Combine first three ingredients and let stand ½ hour. Preheat oven to 350°. Put remaining ingredients on top of oatmeal mixture; stir just until blended. Spoon into 12 large or 36 miniature greased muffin tins. Bake 30–40 minutes or until golden. Turn out onto wire rack to cool slightly before eating. (Makes 12 large or 36 small muffins.)

Quick Bread in the Morning for Busy People

Not a recipe, really. Just a way to have hot bread or muffins even when mornings are rushed.

Medium-size bowl with cover
Large whisk
Large jar with tight lid
Baking pan or muffin tins

When you want to make muffins or quick bread for breakfast, do most of your preparation the night before. Combine all of the dry ingredients for your favorite recipe in a large bowl; blend ingredients well with a large whisk; cover tightly and set aside. Combine all of the liquid ingredients, *except* the egg(s), in a large jar; cover tightly and refrigerate. Wash the egg(s) and leave them out to warm. (If temperature is very warm, refrigerate.) Grease baking pan or line muffin pans with paper liners; set aside. In the morning, simply add the egg to the liquid in the jar; cover, and give it a good shake before pouring over the dry ingredients and blending in lightly with the whisk.

Winter Fruit and Nut Turnovers

You won't be able to resist these! Try having them with herb tea in place of the usual "coffee" break.

2 cups chopped apples
2 cups chopped pears
1½ cups chopped, dried mixed fruit
1 cup apple juice
½ cup honey or maple syrup
Juice and grated rind from ½ lemon
1 tablespoon oil
1 recipe Cheese or Tofu Pastry (page 62)

Combine all ingredients, *except* Cheese Pastry, in a saucepan. Cook for 15 minutes over low heat, stirring occasionally. Allow to cool.

Preheat oven to 425°. Roll out pastry dough to about ⅛-inch thickness. Cut into 3-inch squares or circles. Place a spoonful of filling on one side, fold over pastry and crimp edges. Place on cookie sheets. Bake 15–20 minutes. Cool on wire racks.

Cheese Breakfast Cookies*

These portable apple and cheese pleasers provide a high-protein breakfast that even kids will enjoy.

¾ *cup all-purpose flour*
⅔ *cup butter or margarine, softened*
⅓ *cup firmly packed brown sugar*
1 egg
1 teaspoon vanilla
½ *teaspoon cinnamon*
½ *teaspoon baking powder*
½ *teaspoon salt*
1 ½ cups Quaker Oats (Quick or Old Fashioned, uncooked)
1 cup (4 oz.) shredded Cheddar cheese
¾ *cup raisins*
1 cup peeled, chopped apple

Preheat oven to 375°. Combine flour, butter, sugar, egg, vanilla, cinnamon, baking powder and salt in large bowl; mix well. Add oats, cheese and raisins; mix well. Stir in apple. Drop by heaping tablespoons onto ungreased cookie sheet. Bake 15 minutes or until golden brown. Cool on racks before storing in loosely covered container at room temperature. Makes about 2 dozen cookies.

*Recipe courtesy of The Quaker Oats Company.

Bacony Breakfast Cookies

Bacon, eggs, and orange juice on your way out the door! Try these on a fussy kid!

1 ¼ cups unbleached flour
⅓ *cup brown sugar, firmly packed*
½ *cup Grape-Nuts™ cereal*
½ *pound bacon, cooked, drained, and crumbled*
½ *cup butter or margarine, softened*
1 egg
2 tablespoons frozen orange juice concentrate, undiluted,
    thawed
1 tablespoon grated orange rind

Preheat oven to 350°. Combine dry ingredients; mix well. Add bacon, margarine, egg, orange juice concentrate, and orange rind. Mix until well blended. Drop by level tablespoons 2 inches apart on ungreased cookie sheets. Bake 10–12 minutes or until edges of cookies are lightly browned but cookies are still soft. Makes 2½ dozen.

Take-a-Shake Breakfasts

But don't limit these tasty treats to breakfast only. We've added calorie counts for dieters who want a change from the skinny luncheon sandwich or the canned meal-in-a-glass.

To make each of these nutritious breakfast shakes, start with 2 or 3 crushed ice cubes in your blender. Add the remaining ingredients and blend until frothy and smooth. Pour into pre-chilled thermos. (Add a Breakfast Cookie for a complete breakfast-on-the-go.)

Apple-Almond Shake:
(400 calories)
- ½ cup plain yogurt
- ½ cup apple juice
- ½ cup strawberries
- ¼ cup almonds
- 1 tablespoon maple syrup or honey

B-B-Booster
(225 calories)
- ¾ cup lowfat milk
- 1 small banana, sliced
- 2 rounded tablespoons Kellogg's 40% Protein Concentrate Cereal
- 1 teaspoon honey or sugar

Berry Tasty Shake:
(132 calories)
- ½ cup grapefruit juice
- ½ cup fresh strawberries
- 1 egg white
- 1 tablespoon plain wheat germ
- 1 teaspoon honey or sugar

Golden Eggnog:
(132 calories)
- ¼ cup lowfat milk
- ½ cup orange juice
- 1 egg
- 1 teaspoon honey or sugar

Great Grape:
(163 calories)
- ½ cup grape juice
- ½ cup lowfat yogurt
- 1 egg white
- 1 teaspoon honey

Hi-Pro Shake:
(216 calories)
- 1 6-ounce can pineapple juice
- ½ cup fresh strawberries
- 1 egg white
- 2 rounded tablespoons Kellogg's 40% Protein Concentrate Cereal

Morning Glory:
(210 calories)
- ½ cup orange juice
- 3 medium apricots
- 1 egg
- 1 teaspoon honey

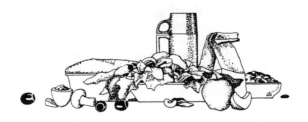

3: Satisfying Sandwiches and Portable Pockets

Yeast Breads and Butters
Nutritious Quick Breads
Sandwich Fillings and Loaves
Sandwich Specials
"Pockets," "Tunnels" and Filled Savories
118 Brown Baggers' Sandwich Combinations

Even before modern man became interested in the nutrient value of the food he ate, he recognized the value of cereal grains in his diet. The early Hebrews either chewed on unleavened matzoth or leavened their bread with sour dough. The bakers for the Egyptian pharaohs mixed their breads with yeasts and enhanced them with herbs, fruits, and honey. Arabs baked their bread in a pancake shape that puffed to form a pocket—just right to stuff with a variety of foods as we do today with that same "modern convenience": pita bread.

It didn't take the invention of the "sandwich," for imaginative cooks to find ways to pack-and-carry their meals. By Shakespeare's time, bread was still the staple food but bakers also prepared "mete pyes and tartes" of pork, game, or lamb "smyte in lytel pecys" and combined with fla-vorful herbs and spices and wrapped in pastry. These hot little packages were just right for feasting on the go.

When you consider that man has packed his meals in neat little pockets since biblical times, you realize (with apologies to the Earl of Sand-wich) that foods don't always have to be carried between two slices of bread. There are sandwiches, pockets, heroes, hoagies, tunnels, savor-ies, pastries, meat pies—the variety is limited only by our imaginations.

Rolled Rye Bread

Oatmeal can be substituted but try the health food department of your supermarket for rolled rye—it has a deliciously robust flavor.

½ cup warm (120°) water
1 package dry yeast
1 tablespoon maple syrup or honey
2 cups cooked rolled rye
2 teaspoons salt
2 tablespoons oil
⅓ cup maple syrup
1½ cups rye flour
2½ cups whole-wheat flour
1 cup unbleached all-purpose flour
½ cup finely chopped walnuts

Mix water, yeast, and 1 tablespoon maple syrup *or* honey in a small bowl; let stand 10–15 minutes. Combine rolled rye, salt, oil, maple syrup, and rye flour in a large bowl; mix in yeast mixture. Beat for 1–3 minutes. Stir in remaining flours and nuts. Turn out onto a floured board or counter and knead until smooth, at least 8–10 minutes. Place in greased bowl, cover and let rise 2 hours. Punch down and form into 2 loaves. Place in greased 9 × 5 × 3-inch pans and let rise 1 hour.

Preheat oven to 400°. Bake 45 minutes or until loaves test done. Turn out onto wire racks to cool.

Light Beer Bread

Makes a nice round slice for bulgur (or beef) burgers.

¼ cup warm (120°) water
1 package dry yeast
2 tablespoons maple syrup or honey
1 egg, slightly beaten
1 teaspoon salt
1 cup warm flat light (or regular) beer
3 cups whole-wheat flour
1½ cups Kellogg's 40% Protein Concentrate Cereal
2 tablespoons oil

Mix water, yeast, and maple syrup *or* honey and let stand while preparing rest of ingredients. Combine remaining ingredients in a large bowl; pour yeast mixture over. Beat well for 1–2 minutes. Spoon batter into 2 greased 1-pound coffee cans; cover with plastic lids. Let rise 1–1¼ hours or until batter is almost touching plastic lids.

Preheat oven to 350°. Remove plastic lids and bake 45–50 minutes or until loaves test done when tried with a cake tester. Cool in cans 10–15 minutes before sliding out onto wire racks to cool. Wrap in foil or plastic wrap to store.

Basic Cornell White Bread

This recipe has been around for years but it still provides extra nutrients for those who prefer a white bread.

3 cups warm water
2 packages active dry yeast
2 tablespoons honey
3 teaspoons salt
2 tablespoons vegetable oil
7–9 cups unbleached flour
½ cup stirred soy flour
3 tablespoons wheat germ
¾ cup nonfat dry milk

Grease 2 9 × 5 × 3-inch bread pans. Combine water, yeast, honey, salt, and oil; let stand 5 minutes to soften yeast. Combine 6 cups of the unbleached flour, soy flour, wheat germ and dry milk. Stir ¾ of the flour mixture into liquid. Beat vigorously, about 75 strokes. Add remaining flour mixture, using your hands if necessary. Dough will be sticky, but will become firmer as you work it. Turn dough onto a floured board; knead, working in as much of remaining flour as is needed to make a smooth dough. Knead 10–15 minutes. Place in oiled bowl, grease the top of the dough lightly and cover with a towel. Allow it to rise in a warm place until doubled, about 1 hour (a fingerprint should remain when dough has risen enough).

Turn onto floured surface and knead briefly. Let rest for 20 minutes. Divide into two portions*, shape into loaves and place in pans. Brush with oil or melted shortening, if desired; cover, and allow breads to rise about 45 minutes.

Preheat oven to 350°. Bake breads 50–60 minutes.

*For smaller loaves, divide into three portions and use 8½ × 4½ × 2½-inch loaf pans. Bake 50 minutes.

Busy Day Tip: You don't have to make yeast bread to take advantage of the extra protein provided by adding "Cornell enrichment formula" to white flour. Any baked goods—quick breads, cookies, cakes—can be fortified in the same manner. Every time you measure 1 cup of flour, simply put 1 tablespoon *each* soy flour, nonfat dry milk, and wheat germ in the bottom of the cup before filling it with flour.

Tabbouleh Bread

The seasonings from the leftover tabbouleh add a wonderful flavor to this bread.

> 2 cups warm (120°) water or *bancha tea*
> ⅓ cup honey or *barley malt syrup*
> 2 packages dry yeast
> ¼ cup oil
> 2 teaspoons salt
> 3 cups whole-wheat flour
> 3 cups unbleached all-purpose flour
> 1 cup cornmeal
> 1 cup uncooked bulgur
> 1½ cups leftover tabbouleh (page 102) drained if necessary

Mix the warm water or tea, 1 tablespoon of the sweetener, and yeast together in a small bowl. Let "proof" while assembling remaining ingredients. Combine oil, salt, remaining sweetener, and whole-wheat flour in a large bowl. Add the yeast mixture. Beat with an electric mixer or wooden spoon 2–3 minutes. Beat in the remaining flours, uncooked bulgur, and tabbouleh, using your hands if necessary. Turn out onto floured board or countertop and knead 2–3 minutes, or until no longer sticky, adding more flour if needed. Place in a greased bowl, cover, and let rise 1–1½ hours or until doubled in size. Punch down. Form into two loaves and place in greased 8 × 4 × 3-inch pans. Let rise 1 hour.

Preheat oven to 375°. Bake 1 hour or until loaves test done. Cool in pan 10–15 minutes before turning out onto wire racks to finish cooling.

Onion Sandwich or Burger Buns

These are wonderful with anything—hamburgers, egg or tuna salad—or just plain.

> 2 cups warm (120°) water
> ¼ cup maple syrup or *barley malt*
> 2 packages dry yeast
> 1 large onion, minced
> ¼ cup corn oil
> ⅛–¼ teaspoon rosemary or *thyme*
> 4 cups wholewheat flour
> 2 cups unbleached all-purpose flour
> 1 teaspoon salt
> sesame or poppy seeds (optional)

Mix hot water and sweetener. Sprinkle yeast into water and let "proof" while preparing onions. Sauté onions in oil until golden, 5–7 minutes, stirring frequently. Stir in yeast mixture, then all of the remaining ingredients. Knead 5–8 minutes; place in greased, covered bowl and let rise until doubled, about 1½ hours. Punch down. Divide into 18 balls and flatten each ball to a 4-inch circle. Place on lightly greased pans. Let rise 1 hour.

Preheat oven to 375°. Lightly brush tops with oil and sprinkle with seeds, if desired. Bake 20–30 minutes.

Ready When You Are Rolls

Unfailingly good—a smooth and supple dough to work with.

2 cups unbleached all-purpose flour
2 packages dry yeast
1 teaspoon salt
2 cups warm (120°) water
¼ cup honey or barley malt
⅓ cup sunflower or corn oil
1 egg (optional)
4 cups whole-wheat flour

Combine the all-purpose flour, yeast, and salt in a large bowl. Stir the honey *or* barley malt and oil into the water; pour over the flour/yeast mixture. Add egg, if using. Beat 3–4 minutes with an electric mixer or wooden spoon. Stir in as much of the whole-wheat flour as you can. Sprinkle remaining flour on a board or countertop. Knead until smooth and elastic, 8–10 minutes. Place in a clean greased bowl, cover and let rise in a warm place until double, about 1½ hours. Punch down dough and let rest, covered, 20 minutes.

Shape into 3 dozen small balls or 12–15 sandwich size rolls and place on lightly greased baking pan. Brush additional oil over the dough shaped rolls; cover pans with plastic wrap or foil; refrigerate. In 3 hours to 3 days, remove from refrigerator. Let rise 45–60 minutes.

Preheat oven to 375°. Bake small rolls for 20 minutes; large rolls 30–40 minutes.

Sandwich Wedge Bread

Great for serving or preparing lunches for a crowd.

> *2 packages dry yeast*
> *½ cup warm (120°) water*
> *1 tablespoon honey*
> *1 cup warm dairy or soy milk (90-100°)*
> *1 cup warm water*
> *¼ cup margarine, softened*
> *6 cups flour (half whole-wheat, if desired)*
> *1 teaspoon salt*

Mix 120° water, honey, and yeast in a large mixing bowl; let "proof" 10 minutes. Stir in milk, water, margarine, salt, and half the flour. Beat with an electric mixer at medium speed for 2 minutes. Stir in the remaining flour with a wooden spoon until well blended, about 2 minutes. Turn into a greased 2-quart casserole. Let rise in a warm spot, covered, about 1-1½ hours until just beginning to rise above casserole.

Preheat oven to 375°. Bake 50–60 minutes. Turn out onto rack to cool.

To serve, slice cooled loaf in half as you would a roll. Layer with your choice of sandwich fillings. Cut into 6–8 pie-shaped wedges.

Butters with Added Punch

Flavored butter can add a wonderful change to the "same old sandwich." Freeze leftovers in small containers for another day.

To ¼ cup of softened butter or margarine, add one of the following:
> *1 teaspoon each wine vinegar and onion juice*
> *1 teaspoon prepared mustard or ¼ teaspoon dry mustard*
> *1 teaspoon Worcestershire sauce*
> *1 tablespoon miso*
> *2 tablespoons finely chopped parsley or chives*
> *½ teaspoon minced onion or garlic*
> *1 teaspoon prepared horseradish*
> *¼ - ½ teaspoon dry or 1 - 1½ teaspoons fresh herb*
>   *(dill, marjoram, oregano, etc.)*
> *½ teaspoon paprika*
> *1 tablespoon honey and 2 tablespoons minced dried apricots*
> *¼ cup flaked tuna*
> *¼ cup minced shrimp*

Appealing Apricot Bread

Great with cream cheese filling.

1¼ cups minced dried apricots
¾ cup water or apple juice
1 cup maple syrup
1 egg, slightly beaten (optional)
2 teaspoons baking powder
½ teaspoon baking soda
2 cups whole-wheat flour
1 cup uncooked oatmeal or rolled rye
1 cup sunflower seeds or chopped almonds

Preheat oven to 350°. Bring water or apple juice and maple syrup to a boil. Pour over apricots and let stand while preparing remaining ingredients. Combine dry ingredients in a medium-size bowl. Stir in egg; pour apricots and liquid over and mix until just blended. Pour into well-greased and floured 9 × 13 × 2-inch pan (or 2 9 × 5 × 3-inch loaf pans). Bake 35–50 minutes or until bread tests done. Let cool in pan 10 minutes before turning out on wire rack to finish cooling.

Whole-Wheat Banana Bread

Like most quick breads, this slices more easily the next day.

1 cup light brown sugar, firmly packed
½ cup soft butter or margarine
2 egg yolks, beaten
2 tablespoons buttermilk or sour milk
1 teaspoon baking soda
1¾ cups whole-wheat flour
½ teaspoon cinnamon
¼ teaspoon salt
1½ cups mashed bananas
½ cup chopped nuts
2 egg whites, beaten until stiff peaks form

Preheat oven to 350°. Cream together sugar and butter; add egg yolks and beat until mixture is light and fluffy. Dissolve baking soda in the buttermilk and add to creamed mixture. Sift together flour, cinnamon, and salt and beat in alternately with bananas just until smooth. Stir in nuts. Fold in stiffly beaten egg whites.

Turn batter into two greased 9 × 5 × 3-inch loaf pans. Bake 1 hour. Cool in pan 10 minutes before turning out onto wire racks to cool. Wrap in foil or plastic wrap to store.

Sweet 'n' Snappy Pear Bread

Take the time to toast the walnuts if you can—it adds a mellow punch to this fragrant bread.

2 cups whole-wheat flour
2 teaspoons baking powder
½ cup chopped walnuts, preferably toasted
1 cup diced fresh pears
¼ cup pear or apple juice
½ cup mild honey
⅓ cup egg or tofu mayonnaise
1 egg
½ teaspoon vanilla extract

Preheat oven to 350°. Combine first three ingredients in bowl. Place remaining ingredients in container of electric blender and blend until smooth. Pour over dry ingredients and mix just until blended. Pour into two greased 8 × 4 × 3-inch loaf pans. Bake 50–60 minutes. Cool in pans 10 minutes before turning out onto wire racks to finish cooling.

Cranberry Banana Bread

2 medium-size ripe bananas
2 cups fresh cranberries
¼ cup oil
½ cup maple syrup
¼ cup honey or ½ cup rice syrup
1½ teaspoons baking powder
½ teaspoon baking soda
2 cups whole-wheat flour (add an additional 2 tablespoons if
    using rice syrup)
1 cup uncooked oatmeal (not instant)

Preheat oven to 350°. Slice bananas into blender. Add whole cranberries, oil, maple syrup, and honey or rice syrup. Chop until cranberries are finely chopped. Combine dry ingredients in a large bowl. Pour blended ingredients over and stir just until blended. Spoon into a 7" × 11" × 2" or 9" × 5" × 3" greased baking pan. Bake 50–60 minutes or until bread tests done. Let cool 10–15 minutes before turning out of pan.

Basic Sandwich Fillings

Egg Salad (1½ cups):
> *4 hard-cooked eggs, chopped*
> *2 tablespoons finely chopped onion or scallions*
> *½ cup finely chopped celery*
> *¼ cup mayonnaise*
> *1 teaspoon prepared mustard*
> *salt and pepper to taste*
> **Substitutions:** *green pepper for celery*
> *sour cream for mayonnaise*
> **Additions:** *Devilled ham, chopped almonds or pimiento*

Ham Salad (1½ cups):
> *1 cup ground or finely chopped fully cooked ham*
> *⅓ cup chopped celery*
> *2 tablespoons pickle relish, drained*
> *½ teaspoon prepared horseradish or mustard*
> *¼ cup mayonnaise*
> **Substitutions:** *canned devilled ham for cooked ham*
> *finely chopped chutney for relish*
> **Additions:** *finely chopped raw carrots, onions, green pepper*

Seafood Salad (1¼ cups):
> *1 6½-ounce can tuna, shrimp, or crab meat, drained and flaked*
> *1 teaspoon lemon juice*
> *¼ cup chopped celery*
> *1 tablespoon minced onion (optional)*
> *3 tablespoons mayonnaise*
> *salt and pepper to taste*
> **Substitutions:** *sweet pickle relish for onions*
> **Additions:** *grated raw carrot*
> *1 tablespoon chili sauce*
> *celery seed to taste*

Chicken Salad (1¼ cups):
> *1 cup finely chopped chicken*
> *¼ cup finely chopped celery*
> *1 tablespoon minced onion or pickle relish*
> *¼ cup mayonnaise*
> **Substitutions:** *chopped pimiento for pickle relish*
> **Additions:** *crumbled bacon or diced ham*

Mix all ingredients thoroughly. Refrigerate.

Sardine Sandwich Filling

If you need an incentive to eat sardines, think of all the calcium they provide.

1 3¾-ounce can sardines
salt and pepper to taste
1 teaspoon lemon juice
1 hard-cooked egg yolk, mashed
3 tablespoons egg or tofu mayonnaise

Drain the oil from the sardines, remove the skins and mash the fish with the salt, pepper, and lemon juice. Mix in egg yolk and mayonnaise. Makes enough filling for two sandwiches.

Add punch to your sandwich by serving with thinly sliced onion on lightly buttered dark bread.

Tuna-Pineapple Spread

Try this on dark rye or pumpernickel bread.

1 6-ounce can white tuna in water, drained
1 8-ounce can crushed pineapple, well drained
¼ cup mayonnaise or crumbled tofu or yogurt
¼ teaspoon salt

Mix ingredients together well. Spread on crackers or use as a filling for 2 sandwiches.

Nutty Chicken Filling

The yogurt and touch of orange make this spread intriguingly appealing.

1 cup cooked minced chicken
½ cup chopped walnuts
¼ cup mayonnaise
¼ cup plain yogurt
1 teaspoon orange juice
¼ teaspoon salt

Mix all ingredients in small bowl. Makes a scant 2 cups or filling for 4 sandwiches.

Add punch to this filling by adding grated orange rind to taste.

Peanut Butter and Tempeh Filling

An excellent way to introduce the nutritional benefits of tempeh to dubious family members.

>1 cup tempeh, ground or finely minced
>½ cup peanut butter
>¼ cup pickle relish (optional)
>2 tablespoons mayonnaise

Mix all ingredients in small bowl. Makes a scant 2 cups of filling.

Egg and Almond Sandwich Filling

Toasted almonds really add punch to this basic egg salad recipe.

>2 hardcooked eggs, minced
>¼ cup almonds, preferably toasted, minced
>¼ cup celery, minced
>¼ – ⅓ cup mayonnaise
>¼ teaspoon salt

Mix all ingredients in small bowl. Makes a heaping ¾ cup.

Beer and Cheese Spread or Stuffing

Can something so easy by so good? Try it and see.

>1 cup beer
>1 pound Cheddar cheese, grated

Put cheese in mixing bowl; pour on beer. Refrigerate, covered, for several hours until cheese has softened. Stir together with a wooden spoon until completely blended. Pack into glass jars or covered containers; store in refrigerator. Lasts at least 2 weeks.

Punched Up Microwave Variation: To the above ingredients in a large mixing bowl, add 1 3-ounce package cream cheese. Microwave at Low for 3–5 minutes. Beat in 3 tablespoons brandy, 1–2 tablespoons oil, 1 teaspoon dry mustard, and 1 teaspoon garlic salt until blended.

Nut Butter

Who needs jelly (and all that sugar)?

>1 cup nuts (peanuts, almonds, or cashews)
>1 tablespoon oil
>Pinch salt

Roast nuts for 20 minutes in a 300° oven, if desired. Cool. Grind in blender, pouring in the oil slowly while the blender is running.

Nut Butter Spread

Sweet and nutritious; try this spread on chappitas, rolled, and sliced into pieces for a quick snack.

1 cup cottage cheese or drained and crumbled tofu
1 cup nut butter
1 tablespoon maple syrup or honey
½ cup chopped dried fruit or raisins

In small bowl, mix ingredients together with a fork. Cover and store in refrigerator. Good on graham crackers or bread.

Add punch to this spread by mixing in 1 tablespoon miso.

Sweet and Spicy Sandwich Spread

This is sweet enough to keep you from being tempted to have dessert instead of a nutritious lunch!

1 apple, washed, cored, and chopped
1 pear, washed, cored, and chopped
¼ cup dates, chopped
¼ cup almonds, chopped
¼ cup peanut or nut butter
¼ teaspoon allspice
1-2 tablespoons apple juice (if needed)

Put all ingredients in blender, adding apple juice if your blender needs it to "move." Whiz just until still somewhat chunky. Try with cream cheese or tofu on graham crackers.

Yogurt Cheese

Try this tasty, low-fat substitute for cream cheese; it will stay fresh in the refrigerator for two weeks.

1 2-pound container plain yogurt, preferably low-fat
Strainer
Cheesecloth, muslin, or clean dish towel

Line a strainer with 2 or 3 thicknesses of cheesecloth, a square of muslin, or a dish towel. Pour in yogurt. Gather edges of fabric at top and secure with a rubber band or tie with a string. Place strainer over a bowl to catch liquid and let stand 6–10 hours at cool room temperature until liquid had drained and "cheese" is thick. (If weather is very warm, place in refrigerator to drain.)

Refrigerate, covered. Makes about 1 cup cheese.

Sloppy Joe Filling

Great to have on hand in the freezer...especially if you have a micro-wave oven at work!

1 pound ground beef
1 medium onion, chopped
1 teaspoon salt
$^1/_8$ teaspoon pepper
2 tablespoons flour
$^1/_2$ teaspoon Worcestershire sauce
$^2/_3$ cup catsup
$^2/_3$ cup water

In large frying pan, brown meat with onion. Stir in salt, pepper, and flour until well blended. Blend in remaining ingredients. Simmer, stirring frequently, 20 minutes, or until thick. Serve on split and toasted hamburger buns. Makes enough filling for 3–4 servings.

To tote, carry hot filling separately in a preheated thermos jar. Easy to pour into a split pita pocket.

Sloppy Jane Filling

Vegetarians can get "sloppy" too!

2 8-ounce packages tempeh
1 large onion, chopped
1 small green pepper, minced
2 tablespoons oil
1 tablespoon tamari or soy sauce
2 tablespoons barley malt or maple syrup
2 tablespoons apple cider vinegar
1 cup spaghetti sauce

Cut tempeh into ½-inch cubes. Sauté the tempeh, onions, and green pepper in the oil for 5 minutes. Stir in remaining ingredients; simmer 20 minutes. Serve on split and toasted whole-wheat hamburger buns or over wide noodles. Makes enough filling for 3–4 servings.

To tote, carry hot filling separately in a preheated thermos jar; pour into a split pita pocket.

Chicken Loaf

Preservative-free, sugar-free, this beats cold cuts any day!

1 pound ground raw chicken or turkey*
1 chicken bouillon cube or 1 teaspoon granules
1 tablespoon minced onion
$^1/_2$ teaspoon salt
$^1/_4$ teaspoon sage
$^1/_4$ teaspoon poultry seasoning
1 teaspoon dried parsley
$^1/_8$ teaspoon pepper
1 slice bread
$^1/_4$ cup hot water
1 egg, slightly beaten
Paprika

Preheat oven to 350°. Break bread slice into crumbs; toss with onion and seasonings in large bowl. Combine water and bouillon; pour over bread and seasonings. Let stand 5 minutes or until bread is softened; mash with fork until bread is finely broken. Add ground chicken or turkey and egg. Mix well. Pack into oiled 8 × 4-inch loaf pan. Sprinkle liberally with paprika. Bake 1 hour, or until meat thermometer registers 175–180°. Delicious hot or cold.

*If grinding the meat yourself, use both light and dark meat. Remove all skin but leave the pockets of fat that are attached to the skin so that loaf will not be too dry. Put through grinder twice.

Ground Beef Meat Loaf

Great for hot or cold for sandwiches, this freezes well.

2 slices whole-wheat or rye bread
2 slices white bread
1 cup water
1 pound lean ground beef
1 medium onion, minced
2 teaspoons dried parsley
1 teaspoon salt
$^1/_4$ teaspoon pepper
1 tablespoon prepared horseradish (optional)
1 egg, slightly beaten
2 tablespoons oil or catsup

Preheat oven to 350°. Pour water over bread in large bowl. When soft, crumble finely with fork. Add remaining ingredients, *except* oil or catsup; mix well. For a crusty loaf, shape into an 8 × 4-inch rectangle and transfer to a shallow baking pan; for a softer exterior, pack into an oiled 8 × 4 × 3-inch loaf pan. Spread top with oil or catsup. Bake 1 hour or until done. Serve hot or chill well before slicing for sandwiches.

Vary by substituting ⅛ teaspoon *each* basil, oregano, and thyme for horseradish and ½ cup tomato juice for part of the water. Handy to have for slicing and adding to quick pita or English muffin pizza snacks.

Tuna-Tofu Loaf

Prepare this in the morning to bake for lunch or dinner; use the leftovers for luncheon sandwiches the next day.

1 6½-ounce can tuna, drained
3 eggs, slightly beaten*
¼ cup dry bread crumbs
1 small onion, minced
1 tablespoon dried parsley
½ cup tomato sauce
½ teaspoon salt
½ teaspoon baking powder
1 cup tofu (about ¼ pound)

Press tofu to remove excess moisture. Crumble and measure; place on paper towel to drain any additional moisture while preparing remaining ingredients. In mixing bowl, flake tuna and combine with remaining ingredients *except* tofu. Fold in tofu gently but thoroughly. Pour into greased 8 × 4 × 3-inch loaf pan, cover, and refrigerate for at least 1 hour (but no longer than 1 day).

Preheat oven to 350°. Bake, uncovered, for 50–60 minutes or until brown.

*An additional ¾ cup tofu may be substituted for the eggs to please non-egg eaters in your family.

Golden Garbanzo Loaf

This isn't the usual heavy bean loaf but a light, golden loaf that is good hot or cold.

1 15-ounce can chick peas, drained
1 large onion, grated
1 stalk celery, grated
½ red or green pepper, grated
2 tablespoons oil
2 tablespoons white wine or apple juice
1 cup soft bread crumbs
¾ cup orange or pineapple juice
¾ cup grated Parmesan cheese
1 egg
½ teaspoon salt
¼ teaspoon Tabasco sauce

Preheat oven to 375°. Chop or mash chick peas. Sauté the vegetables in the oil and wine or apple juice for several minutes on high heat. Mix in all remaining ingredients and spoon into a greased 8 × 4-inch bread pan. Bake 45–50 minutes. Good hot or cold.

Great Grain Loaf

Good hot, warm, or cold.

2 cups cooked grain (rice, barley, millet, etc.)
4 eggs, lightly beaten
1 cup grated or minced carrots
1-2 cups grated Cheddar or Swiss cheese
½ cup plain yogurt or sour cream
½ cup minced scallions or ¼ cup minced onion
½ teaspoon salt
¼ teaspoon pepper
¼ teaspoon ground cumin (optional)

Preheat oven to 350°. Mix all ingredients together well. Spoon into greased 8 × 4-inch bread pan; smooth top. Set into a larger pan which you have half filled with hot water. Bake 65 minutes or until a knife inserted in the center comes out clean. Let stand 15 minutes before turning out and slicing.

Oven Baked Turkey Meatballs

Delicious hot or cold, with or without a sauce.

> 1 pound ground turkey
> 1 medium onion, grated or minced
> 1 large stalk celery, grated or minced
> ²/₃ cup fresh bread crumbs or cooked rice
> 1 tablespoon oil
> ¹/₄ cup water or apple juice
> ¹/₈ teaspoon nutmeg (optional)
> ¹/₂ teaspoon poultry seasoning

Preheat oven to 375°. Mix all ingredients together well and form into balls 1–1½-inch in diameter. Place on greased cookie sheet. Bake 45 minutes or until browned. Good plain or with spaghetti sauce.

To tote, pack hot meatballs and sauce in preheated wide mouth thermos and carry a grinder roll separately. Or, stuff cold meatballs into pita bread with zucchini or cucumber slices and a thin slice of Swiss cheese.

My Hero!

> *"Hero" rolls*
> *Prosciutto ham*
> *Capicola or Genoa salami*
> *Provolone cheese*
> *Romano cheese, grated (optional)*
> *Italian olive salad, drained*

Split and butter rolls or spread lightly with olive oil. Fill sandwich with layers of meats and cheeses; top with olive salad. (To make several sandwiches at once, substitute a large loaf of French or Italian bread; cut loaf into thick slices.)

To tote, prepare sandwich as directed *except* carry Italian olive salad separately in a small container. Add to sandwich just before eating.

Tunnel Sandwiches

Easy for small hands to hold and eat.

> *Unsplit hero or hot dog rolls*
> *Tuna, egg, or chicken salad filling*

With fork, hollow out the center of the roll, forming a "tunnel" but leaving a firm shell. (Save the removed crumbs and dry for use in meat loaf or as a casserole topping.) Stuff with desired filling and wrap tightly in foil or plastic wrap.

French Loaf Special

This super recipe is from the Campbell Soup Company.

2 5-ounce cans chunk style mixin' chicken
1 cup shredded Cheddar cheese
½ cup mayonnaise
¼ cup chopped pimiento-stuffed olives
2 tablespoons sweet pickle relish
French bread (approximately 17-inches long)

In bowl, combine all ingredients except bread. Cut bread in half lengthwise to within ½ inch of side. Hollow out each half, leaving a shell ½-inch thick. Fill each shell with chicken mixture. Fold bread together; wrap in foil. Chill overnight. Cut loaf into 4 slices.

Pita with Ham Almond Filling

Nice in pita; just as good with dark bread.

3 cups finely chopped cooked ham
½ cup chopped toasted almonds
⅓ cup sliced scallions
1 3-ounce package cream cheese, softened
½ cup mayonnaise

In bowl, combine all ingredients well. Enough to fill 3 pita pockets.

Stuffed Pita Pockets

Neat to eat; no more filling oozing out between the slices of bread!

½ cup bulgur
1 cup boiling water
¼ cup raisins
1 cup shredded carrot
¼ cup sunflower seeds
Whole-wheat pita bread
Lettuce

Pour boiling water over bulgur in medium size bowl. Cover and let stand 30 minutes or until soft. Drain well. Stir in raisins, carrots, and sunflower seeds. Cover and chill. When ready to prepare sandwiches, stir in yogurt. Cut large pita rounds in half crosswise or slit medium-size rounds at one edge and open. Line with lettuce leaves and spoon about ⅓ cup mixture into each.

Stuffed Pita with Salad

Especially good with thinly sliced ham and cheese.

Pita bread
Sliced meat, cheese, seafood, and/or grains
2 cups shredded lettuce
1 small tomato, peeled and diced
1 tablespoon minced onion
¼ cup mayonnaise
3 tablespoons wine vinegar
½ teaspoon salad herb mixture
¼ teaspoon oregano (or to taste)
Salt and pepper to taste
Alfalfa sprouts

Stuff pita bread with favorite combination of meat, cheese, seafood, and/or grains. Combine remaining ingredients, *except* alfalfa sprouts and pile on top. Sprinkle with alfalfa sprouts. Makes enough salad for 3–4 sandwiches.

To package, stuff pita with fillings and sprinkle with alfalfa sprouts; wrap in foil or plastic wrap. Carry salad mixture in separate small container; pile on top just before eating.

Bulgur Burgers

These are good cold or at room temperature and they stay crisp even when packed-to-go.

1 cup reconstituted or cooked bulgur
1 onion, minced
1 stalk celery, minced
1 clove garlic, minced
½ cup almond butter
¼ cup ground almonds
2 tablespoons water or lemon juice
¼ cup whole-wheat flour
½ teaspoon salt
2 tablespoons each oil and tamari or soy sauce

Combine all ingredients, *except* oil and tamari, until well blended. Form into ¼–½-inch thick patties. Heat the oil and tamari sauce in a large frying pan. Sauté several minutes until crisp and golden. Turn and repeat for remaining sides.

To package, make ahead and chill separately before placing in roll or between slices of bread spread with flavored butter.

Greenwiches

Sophisticated and slightly spicy...try as a cocktail tidbit, too.

> $1/4$ *cup tofu or cottage cheese, drained and crumbled*
> *1 3-ounce package cream cheese, softened*
> *2 bunches watercress, stems removed*
> $1/4$ *teaspoon salt*
> $1/8$ *teaspoon rosemary*

Place ingredients in blender and blend until smooth. Good on sourdough rye bread or rye crackers.

Chicken and Eggwiches

Can't make up your mind what to have? Try this.

> *1 cup minced cooked chicken*
> *1 cup minced hard-cooked eggs*
> *⅓ cup egg or tofu mayonnaise*
> *1 teaspoon lemon juice*
> *1 teaspoon prepared mustard*
> *1 teaspoon tamari or soy sauce*

Combine ingredients. Serve on crackers or use as a sandwich filling.

Spanish Eggs in Crepes

No time to make crêpes? These eggs are just as good served stuffed into warmed pita bread.

> *8 whole-wheat or cornmeal crepes*
> *8 eggs, well beaten*
> *½ cup chopped mushrooms*
> *½ cup minced red or green pepper*
> *2 tablespoons chopped canned green chilis (optional)*
> *½ cup minced onion*
> *1 8-ounce can mild taco sauce*
> *¼ teaspoon salt*
> *1 cup grated Monterey Jack cheese (optional)*
> *1 tablespoon oil*
> *2 tablespoons margarine*

Preheat oven to 450°. In large frying pan, sauté mushrooms, pepper, and onion in oil over high heat, 4–5 minutes, stirring constantly. Lower heat; add margarine. When margarine is melted, add eggs and cook, stirring gently, until just done. Add green chilis.

Spoon filling onto crepes. Roll up and place in greased baking dish. Pour on taco sauce. Sprinkle with cheese, if desired. Bake 10 minutes.

Chicken and Tomatoes in Pita

3 chicken breast fillets
1 cup cherry tomatoes, halved
1 tablespoon oil
1 clove garlic, minced
1 tablespoon lemon juice or white wine
2 tablespoons minced parsley or chives

Preheat oven to 400°. Cut chicken into 1-inch cubes; toss with all remaining ingredients. Place in 1-quart casserole and bake 20 minutes. Stuff into warmed pita bread. Makes enough to fill 6 medium or 3 large pita pockets split in half.

Pastries for Portable Pockets

Quick and Easy Pastry:

2 cups unbleached all-purpose or 1 ¾ cups whole-wheat flour
¼ teaspoon salt
⅔ cup mayonnaise
2 tablespoons cold water

Stir the flour and salt together in a mixing bowl. In a separate small bowl, combine the mayonnaise and water; then mix into the flour and salt with a fork just until the dough gathers into a ball. Makes two 9-inch pie crusts or can be used for tarts or turnovers.

Yogurt Pastry:

1 cup margarine, melted
½ teaspoon salt
1 cup plain yogurt
2 cups whole-wheat or 2 ¼ cups all-purpose flour

Mix ingredients until a ball forms. Chill in freezer for one-half hour. Roll out on pastry cloth or waxed paper. Makes 12–16 (double crust) 4-inch "pielets."

Cheese or Tofu Pastry:

1 cup margarine or ½ cup margarine and ⅓ cup oil
1 cup cottage cheese or well-drained, crumbled tofu
2 cups sifted whole-wheat flour
1 tablespoon honey
¼ teaspoon salt

Cream margarine, honey, and cream cheese or tofu together until smooth and creamy. Sift together remaining ingredients. Work into creamed mixture with a pastry cutter or wooden spoon until completely blended in. Form into a ball; wrap in plastic wrap and chill several hours in refrigerator. Use as directed for pie shells or turnovers.

Vegetable Tartlets Italiano

Good hot for lunch at home or cold in the lunch box.

1 recipe Yogurt Pastry (page 61)
½ cup minced onion
½ cup minced green pepper
2 tablespoons oil, preferably olive oil
1 cup chick peas, mashed
1 cup minced zucchini
1 8-ounce can tomato sauce
1 teaspoon oregano
¼ teaspoon thyme
¼ teaspoon rosemary
½ teaspoon salt

Preheat oven to 400°. In small frying pan, sauté the onion and pepper in the oil for 5 minutes. Add the remaining ingredients; simmer, uncovered, 5 minutes. Cool to room temperature. Meanwhile, roll pastry ⅛–¼-inch thick and cut into desired shapes. Spoon filling by heaping tablespoons in center of 4-inch pastry rounds; cover with additional pastry rounds and crimp edges. (For smaller tartlets, use 4-inch pastry squares and fold over to form a triangle.) Place on lightly greased cookie sheets. Bake 18–20 minutes. Makes 12–16 tartlets.

Mini-Meat Pies

1 recipe Cheese Pastry (page 61)
½ pound lean ground beef
1 small onion, chopped
½ teaspoon salt
¼ teaspoon marjoram
1 teaspoon dried parsley
Pepper to taste
1 tablespoon dry bread crumbs (if needed)

Preheat oven to 425°. In frying pan, brown meat with onion. Add remaining ingredients (including bread crumbs if filling is very moist). Allow to cool while rolling pastry to about ⅛" thickness. Cut rolled pastry into 4" squares; place about 1 tablespoon filling on each. Fold in half diagonally and press edges with tines of fork to seal. Place pies on lightly greased cookie sheets and bake 15 minutes or until lightly browned.

To tote, cool completely before wrapping or placing in sandwich container.

New Style Reubens

Double the recipe if desired. Try these with Very Vegetable Soup!

½ recipe Yogurt Pastry (page 61)
½ cup minced turkey
½ cup minced ham
¼ cup shredded Swiss cheese
1 tablespoon minced pickle relish
2 tablespoons sauerkraut (optional)
1 teaspoon Dijon mustard
2 tablespoons plain yogurt or sour cream

Preheat oven to 400°. Combine all ingredients and mix well. Spoon on 4-inch pastry squares by heaping tablespoonfuls. Fold pastry over to form a triangle; crimp edges with tines of fork to seal. Place on lightly greased cookie sheets. Bake 18–20 minutes. Makes 1–1½ dozen.

Tuna Tempters

Much more exciting than the old "tuna-on-rye."

1 recipe Cheese Pastry (page 61)
1 6½-ounce can tuna, drained
1 cup minced raw cauliflower
½ cup minced celery
1 cup shredded Cheddar or Swiss cheese
½ cup egg or tofu mayonnaise
⅛ teaspoon Tabasco sauce
¼ teaspoon salt

Preheat oven to 350°. Roll pastry and cut into 4-inch rounds or squares. Combine remaining ingredients and spoon 2 level tablespoons onto center of each turnover; fold over and crimp edges with tines of fork to seal. Place on lightly greased cookie sheets. Bake 25 minutes or until golden.

Busy Day Variation: Add ½ cup grated Cheddar or other firm cheese and 2 tablespoons minced olives to ½ cup leftover tuna salad. Make 12 turnovers, using only half recipe Cheese Pastry. [Use the other half of the pastry for *Jim Jams* (page 141) or *Apple Turnovers* (page 141).]

Onion Turnovers

If you're an onion lover, you'll devour these with pleasure.

1 recipe favorite pastry
3 onions, minced
½ cup margarine
1 cup plain yogurt or sour cream
1 egg
½ teaspoon salt

Preheat oven to 400°. In small frying pan, sauté the onions in the margarine until golden. Remove from heat; stir in remaining ingredients. Spoon heaping tablespoonfuls onto 3-inch pastry squares. Fold over to form triangle and crimp edges with tines of fork to seal. Bake 15 minutes. Good hot, cold, or at room temperature.

Green Bean Packages

Garden overflowing with beans? These are wonderfully light and delicate.

1 recipe Yogurt Pastry (page 61)
2½ cups fresh green beans, snipped into ¼-inch pieces
1 small onion, minced
1–2 cloves garlic, minced
1 tablespoon tahini
2 tablespoons mayonnaise
½ teaspoon salt

Preheat oven to 400°. Cook the green beans and onion in a small amount of boiling water until tender, about 10–12 minutes. Drain well. Combine with remaining ingredients. Spoon heaping tablespoons onto 4-inch pastry rounds. Cover with additional pastry rounds; crimp edges with tines of fork to seal. Place on lightly greased cookie sheets. Bake 18–20 minutes or until golden. Makes 12–16 "pielets." Good eating cold or at room temperature.

SANDWICHES THAT SATISFY

Some Like 'Em Hot

To reheat: For reheating in a conventional oven, tote sandwich securely wrapped in foil. Most sandwiches heat up in 10–15 minutes in a 375° oven. For reheating in microwave oven, tote sandwich wrapped in plastic wrap or waxed paper. To reheat, place unwrapped sandwich on paper plate and cover with paper towel or napkin. Reheat at Medium power level for 1–2 minutes or to a serving temperature of 110°. If sandwich is frozen, increase time by about one-half.

Barbecued Beef* in pita bread (carried separately or reheated)
Beans (mashed) with minced onion and Worcestershire sauce added—
  American cheese—mustard butter—whole-wheat roll* or thickly
  sliced Italian bread—heat until filling is hot and cheese melts
Cheese—crisp bacon—tomato—mustard butter—whole-wheat roll*—
  heat until cheese melts
Cheese—drained leftover Ratatouille—butter—whole wheat bun*
Cheese filling (½ c. grated American cheese combined with 1 T. cat-
  sup, 1 t. mustard, 1 t. instant minced onion)—2 hamburger buns—
  heat until cheese melts
Corned Beef Reubens*—pumpernickel rolls or whole-wheat buns
Corned beef—mustard butter—sliced dill pickle—rye bread
Corned beef—Swiss cheese—sauerkraut—Thousand Island dressing—
  rye or pumpernickel bread—heat just until cheese is melted
Ham Salad* with diced Cheddar cheese and minced dill pickle added
  stuffed into hollowed out frankfurter roll—heat until cheese melts
Ham (baked or boiled)—mozzarella cheese—cooked turkey—blue
  cheese or butter—grinder roll—heat until cheese melts
Ham (boiled)—sliced tomato—sliced dill pickle—crumbled Roquefort
  or blue cheese (instead of butter)—(bake at 425°)
Ham (boiled)—Swiss cheese—butter—rye bread
Roast beef—Swiss cheese—poppy seed flavored butter*—hard roll—
  1½ minutes or until rolls warm
Salami—Swiss cheese or Monterey Jack—Flavored Butter*—rye rolls
Sloppy Joe filling* in pita bread (carried separately or reheated)
Tuna Tempters filling* on whole-wheat hamburger bun—heat until
  rolls are hot and cheese is melted.
Turkey—Ham—Cheese

Some Like 'Em Cold

Remember: the basic rules for preventing soggy sandwiches if you are preparing any of these ahead of time.

Bacon (crisp slices)—blue cheese and cream cheese combined with horseradish, onion, and a dash of Worcestershire—tomato slices—lettuce—mayonnaise—white bread

Beans (mashed) mixed with a bit of minced onion and chili sauce—butter—pumpernickel bread

Beans (mashed)—chili sauce—pickle relish—butter—rye bread

Beans—thinly sliced onion—chili sauce—whole-wheat bread

Braunschweiger or liverwurst—Swiss or other cheese—mustard butter—French bread or whole wheat roll*

Cheese (Monterey Jack)—shredded lettuce—sliced tomato—mayonnaise thinned with barbecue sauce and spiced with garlic

Cheese filling*—rye bread or chappati

Cheese (Swiss or Provolone)—well drained leftover Ratatouille or Eggplant Parmesan—pita bread

Cheese (Ricotta) with minced hard cooked egg and grated carrot added—dark bread

Chicken loaf*—flavored butter*—rye bread

Chicken salad*—ham (boiled) or bacon—stuffed into pita bread

Chicken salad* with diced ham and green pepper added—rye bread

Chicken salad* with diced apple or pineapple added—pita bread

Chicken—bacon slices—blue cheese—whole-wheat or white bread

Chicken—bacon—tomato—mustard butter—whole-wheat bread

Chicken—ham (boiled)—Swiss cheese—cole slaw

Chicken—pineapple—lettuce—mayonnaise

Chick pea Salad (Hummus)*—mayonnaise—pita bread

Chili Bean Dip* in pita bread

Corned beef—pastrami—whole-wheat bun*

Corned beef—Swiss cheese—sauerkraut—mustard butter—rye bread

Cottage cheese mixed with chopped dried apricots and nuts or seeds—whole-wheat bread

Cottage cheese mixed with chopped onion, green pepper, carrot, and/or celery—whole-wheat bread

Cream cheese mixed with pineapple and nuts—rye bread

Cream cheese (or cottage cheese) combined with marmalade or grated orange rind and finely chopped nuts—dark bread or nut bread

Cream cheese blended with crushed strawberries or peaches—rye or Sweet 'n' Snappy Pear Bread*

Cream cheese—Appealing Apricot Bread*

Cream cheese—crushed pineapple—Cranberry Banana Bread*

Cream cheese—dried chipped beef—rye bread
Cream cheese—marmalade or jelly—rye bread or Rolled Rye Bread*
Cream cheese—olives—pimiento—whole-grain bread
Cream cheese—nuts—raisins—whole-wheat or Boston Brown Bread
Cream cheese—tart jam (like currant)—rye bread
Cream cheese—thinly sliced cucumber and green pepper and/or onion
 —lettuce—mayonnaise—rye bread
Cream cheese—thinly sliced smoked salmon—thinly sliced sweet onion
 —butter—dark rye bread or bagels
Duck (thinly sliced)—tart marmalade—butter—rye bread
Egg salad*—lettuce—butter—any bread or whole-wheat pita
Egg salad* mixed with cottage cheese or tofu
Egg salad* with bacon, devilled ham, or minced boiled ham and pickle
 relish added—rye bread
Egg—sliced tomato—alfalfa sprouts—lettuce—mayonnaise
Ham salad*—Swiss cheese—sliced tomato—rye bread
Ham salad*—thinly sliced Cheddar cheese—rye bread
Ham (baked or boiled)—pineapple—green pepper rings—lettuce—
 mayonnaise
Ham (baked)—Swiss cheese—chicken—hard-cooked egg slices—
 romaine lettuce—tomato or thinly sliced onion—hard roll or baked
 brown-and-serve French bread
Ham (baked)—turkey—Swiss cheese—cole slaw
Ham (prosciutto)—Genoa salami—provolone cheese—lettuce—
 mustard—mayonnaise—hero roll
Ham (ground) mixed with orange or pineapple and mustard—mayon-
 naise—dark bread
Liverwurst—lettuce—tomato—mustard butter—whole-wheat bread
Liverwurst—thinly sliced red onion—sliced cucumber—lettuce—
 butter mixed with horseradish—dark rye bread
Liverwurst—thinly sliced sharp Cheddar cheese—thinly sliced tomato
 —sliced red onion—rye bread
Lobster salad—hero roll hollowed out to make a Tunnel Sandwich*
Luncheon meat—green pepper rings—lettuce—onion roll
Meat loaf*—chili sauce—favorite bread
Nut butters: see combinations listed under "peanut butter"
Pastrami—provolone cheese—lettuce—tomato—blue cheese dressing
 —butter—rye bread
Peanut butter mixed with chopped raisins and and grated carrots or
 crushed pineapple—whole-wheat bread
Peanut butter and sautéed onion blended until creamy—whole-wheat
 bread
Peanut butter mixed with honey and chopped nuts or dates—whole-
 wheat bread or chappati

Peanut butter—bacon—whole-wheat bun*
Peanut butter—honey—sunflower seeds—whole-wheat bread
Peanut butter—orange marmalade—rye bread
Peanut butter—thin slices of apple—whole-wheat bread
Roast beef (ground) and mixed with chopped pickle and celery, prepared horseradish, and mayonnaise—rye bread
Roast beef—chili sauce—whole-wheat bread
Roast beef—horseradish flavored mustard—lettuce—pumpernickel
Roast beef—Roquefort cheese—Worcestershire flavored butter*—rye bread
Salmon Seafood Salad* with minced cucumber added
Salmon—cream cheese—pumpernickel
Sardine filling*—mustard or tuna butter—pumpernickel bread
Sardine or kipper snacks—sliced hard-cooked egg—sliced cucumber—sliced tomato—hard roll
Sardine—sliced onion—mustard—pumpernickel bread
Sardine—Swiss cheese—sliced onion—tomato—rye bread
Seafood Salad* (substitute 1 cup shredded leftover cooked fillet of fish)—lettuce—mayonnaise—whole-wheat bread
Shrimp Seafood Salad*—green pepper rings—lettuce—rye bread
Shrimp—thinly sliced cucumber—butter—rye bread
Tabbouleh* (well drained)—pita bread
Tofu Egg Salad (substitute ½ cup well drained crumbled tofu for two of the eggs in Egg Salad*)—mayonnaise—whole-wheat bread
Tongue—Swiss cheese—lettuce—rye bread
Tongue—Swiss cheese—sliced gherkins—butter—whole-wheat bread
Tuna Salad*—hard boiled egg—tomato—mayonnaise—whole-wheat bun
Tuna Salad* with diced Swiss cheese mixed in—Onion Sandwich Bun*
Tuna Salad*—spinach leaves—pumpernickel
Tuna Salad* with raisins and a dash of curry powder added
Tuna-Apple—add 1 diced small apple to Tuna Salad*—pita bread
Tuna-Tofu Loaf*—chili sauce—rye bread
Turkey—beef tongue—Swiss cheese—coleslaw—Thousand Island Dressing—rye bread
Turkey—cranberry sauce—lettuce—mayonnaise—rye bread
Turkey—pastrami—mustard or herb butter—rye bread
Turkey—sliced hard-cooked egg—sliced tomato—Russian Dressing—whole-wheat bread
Turkey—tongue—cole slaw—rye bread
Vegetable loaf or Golden Garbanzo Loaf*—sliced tomatoes—lettuce—mayonnaise—dark bread

*See index for recipe

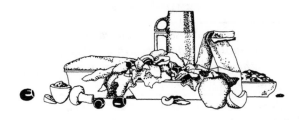

4: Super Soups and Stews

Soup Starters
Hot Soups and Stews
Cold Soups
Canned and Instant Soups

History tells us that the soup ladle was invented by the Duc de Montausier about 1695. However, historical references to soup go as far back as 2000 B.C. when Indian Vedic literature mentioned parched barley ground up with juices. Later, the Greeks flavored their barley "soup" with aromatic herbs like mint, pennyroyal, or thyme and it served as a ritual beverage at the mysteries of Eleusis. The first-century Roman writer, Apicius, mentions a barley soup with lentils, peas, and chick peas.

In early times, soup was called *pottage* (from the Latin *potare*, to drink). In Medieval times it became customary to dunk hunks of bread, called *sop*, in the stew broth. Eventually the word was applied to the broth itself. In time it became our modern word, *soup*.

With instinctive wisdom, our ancestors were tending to their nutritional needs. Today, we appreciate that one of the greatest values of soup is that it retains all the vitamins, particularly the fat-soluble vitamins A, D, and E, which are often lost (or drained away) in cooking other foods. Soups are also more apt to contain a balanced variety of protein-rich ingredients—especially meat, beans, poultry or fish.

For lunch toters who have access to a wide variety of insulated carrying containers, soups and stews offer the ideal way to pack a nutritionally balanced meal in one container.

[69]

Soup Starter

When you make your own soups, you can control the amount of sodium, fat, and additives more easily than when you use commercial soups. Keep a supply of soup stock in your freezer to add flavor and nutrients to your home made soups.

5 pounds meaty chicken* or beef bones* or 4 cups fresh or leftover vegetables*
2 celery stalks with tops, sliced
2 medium onions, chopped
2 carrots, chopped
1 bay leaf
¼ teaspoon thyme
1 tablespoon dried parsley

Place bones and/or vegetables in large kettle; add cold water to cover. Bring to boil, skimming off foam as it rises to surface. Bring to boil; reduce heat, cover, and simmer chicken or beef stock 3–4 hours or vegetable stock 30 minutes or until vegetables are soft. Strain and discard solids. Cool broth quickly; refrigerate until any fat is solid. Remove and discard hardened fat.

*Use chicken wings, backs, necks, giblets, or bones saved from making your own chicken "cutlets." Try to get a few marrow bones, sawed in pieces, to add extra flavor to beef stock. Fresh or leftover green beans, turnips, lettuce, tomatoes, and/or parsnips all add flavor to vegetable stock; yellow or zucchini squash adds a sweet flavor as well as valuable potassium to the stock.

Lunch in a Mug: Soup

This "almost instant" soup recipe from Republic Molding Corporation (the makers of the Micro-Mug) is a boon at home or at the office. If you have a microwave oven at work, keep a jar of this in your desk drawer or locker.

¾ cup non-fat dry milk powder
¼ cup non-dairy creamer
2 tablespoons instant chicken bouillon granules
1 tablespoon dried vegetable flakes
½ teaspoon dried parsley flakes
½ teaspoon dried summer savory
½ teaspoon salt
¼ teaspoon onion powder
¼ teaspoon pepper
Instant rice (optional)

In a small bowl combine all dry ingredients, *except* rice. Store in airtight container no longer than 6 months.

To serve 1: Place 2 tablespoons instant rice and 3 tablespoons dry soup mix in the Micro-Mug. Stir in ¾ cup water and microwave at High 1½ to 3 minutes, or until boiling; stir. Cover with plastic wrap and let stand 5 minutes, or until rice is tender.

To serve 2: Place ¼ cup instant rice and ⅓ cup dry soup mix in the Micro-Mug. Stir in 1½ cups water and microwave at High 3 to 4 minutes, or until boiling; stir. Cover and let stand 5 minutes, or until rice is tender.

Creamy Mushroom Soup

This really is creamy...you won't miss the milk.

> *1 pound mushrooms, sliced*
> *2 cloves garlic, minced*
> *1 onion, minced*
> *¼ cup oil*
> *4 cups water*
> *1½ cups almonds or cashews**
> *2 tablespoons miso*
> *Fresh dillweed (optional)*

Sauté mushrooms, garlic, and onion in oil until golden. Meanwhile, place remaining ingredients in blender and blend until smooth. Pour over mushrooms. Simmer gently, 20–30 minutes. Sprinkle with minced fresh dill, if desired.

*If the price of almonds or cashews makes you shudder at the dent in your budget, substitute 4 cups milk for the water and nuts.

Tomato Rice Soup

A beautiful soup...especially good with cornbread.

> *3–4 cloves garlic, minced*
> *1 tablespoon oil*
> *5–6 garden tomatoes, peeled and coarsely chopped*
> *2 quarts vegetable stock*
> *¾ cup cooked brown rice*
> *½–1 teaspoon dill or thyme*

Sauté garlic in oil, stirring constantly, until golden. Add remaining ingredients and simmer 10–15 minutes.

Add punch by using tamari sauce instead of oil to sauté the garlic. (Saves calories, too!)

Very Vegetable Soup

This is our all-time favorite vegetable soup. Security is having a potful in the freezer or fridge!

1 medium onion, chopped
1 clove garlic, minced
3 medium carrots, diced
2 tablespoons oil
4 cups water or vegetable stock (3 cups if you like a thick soup)
1 1-pound can tomatoes
⅔ cup each: cut green beans
              diced celery
              shredded cabbage or *cauliflower*
1 small zucchini, diced
1 tablespoon dried parsley
1 bay leaf
Salt and pepper to taste

Sauté onion and garlic in oil until tender crisp; add carrots and continue to cook for another minute or until carrots are coated with oil. (To bring out the flavor of the vegetables, sprinkle about ½ teaspoon sugar over the carrots as you cook and stir.) Add remaining ingredients. Bring to boil; lower heat; simmer 45 minutes or until all vegetables are tender.

Potato Soup

Cold weather appetites respond to this flavorful soup!

2 pounds white or sweet potatoes, pared and sliced
1 onion, peeled and thinly sliced
1 carrot, minced
1 celery stalk, minced
¼ cup oil
1 quart vegetable or chicken broth
¼ cup chopped chives or *fresh parsley*
Paprika
Grated Parmesan, Swiss, or *Cheddar cheese (optional)*

Steam potatoes until very tender. Drain and mash or put through a ricer. Sauté onion, carrot, and celery in oil, about 5 minutes or until barely tender. Stir in potatoes until blended. Stir in broth and simmer several minutes. Spoon into bowls and sprinkle with chives or parsley, paprika, and cheese.

To tote, pour into preheated thermos and sprinkle with cheese.

Add Punch by stirring in 1 can tuna (drained) to make a hearty chowder.

Busy Day Variation: In saucepan, blend together and heat, stirring occasionally: 1 10¾-ounce can condensed Cream-of-Potato Soup, ⅛ teaspoon dry mustard, 1 soup can milk, ½ cup shredded Swiss cheese, and 2 tablespoons chopped parsley.

To serve cold: (Vichysoisse) Use white potatoes, preferably baking potatoes. Reduce chicken broth to 3 cups. After cooking as directed, cool slightly before blending in electric blender. Stir in 2 cups milk and/or cream; adjust seasonings and chill well.

Quick Clam Chowder

This is almost as fast as opening a can—and much tastier.

1 small onion, chopped
1 small clove garlic, minced
½ small green pepper, chopped
1 medium carrot, diced
2 tablespoons oil or margarine
1 tomato, peeled and chopped
1 large stalk celery, diced
1 large potato, diced
1 cup chicken broth
2 cups water
1 small bayleaf
⅛ teaspoon thyme
1 8-ounce can minced clams (broth included)

Sauté onion, garlic, green pepper, and carrot in oil or margarine until onion is golden and slightly tender. Add chicken broth and water; add remaining ingredients, *except* clams. Simmer 15 minutes or until vegetables are tender. Add clams and broth. Reheat.

Chicken Noodle Soup-to-Go

This soup "cooks" in the thermos.

1 cup chicken broth
1 tablespoon each: minced celery
minced onion
minced red pepper
¼ teaspoon thyme
3 tablespoons uncooked alphabet or fine noodles

Bring broth to a boil. Combine remaining ingredients in thermos. Pour broth over; cap tightly, shake, and let stand 30 minutes or longer.

Red Lentil Soup

Try this for the holiday season—or Valentine's Day!

½-pound kale, spinach, or mustard greens
1 large onion, coarsely chopped
1 red pepper, cut in thin strips
¼ cup oil
1½ cups vegetable stock
1 cup cooked red lentils
Juice of 1 lemon
1 teaspoon grated lemon rind

Wash and shred greens; drain well. Sauté onion and red pepper for 5 minutes in the oil. Add greens and sauté until greens are coated with oil. Add stock and lentils. Simmer 20–30 minutes. Stir in lemon juice and rind. Serve hot.

Beef Barley Soup

This is a robust soup to bring cheer to a cold winter day. Make enough to freeze some, too.

2 pounds meaty beef soup bones
2 quarts water or beef broth
1 tablespoon dried parsley
1 teaspoon salt (or to taste)
¼ teaspoon pepper
½ cup barley, rinsed
½ cup chopped onion
½ cup chopped celery
½ cup diced carrots
1 16-ounce can tomatoes
1 cup fresh or frozen peas or cut string beans

Remove meat from bones; cube the meat and brown meat and bones (adding a small amount of oil, if necessary). Add water or broth, parsley, and salt and pepper. Simmer one hour; add barley and cook for another hour. Remove bones from soup; skim off any excess fat. Add onion, celery, carrots, and tomatoes; cook 45 minutes. Add peas or string beans; cook 15 minutes longer.

Busy Day Variation: In small saucepan, brown 1 cup cubed leftover cooked beef or ham in 1 tablespoon melted butter. Add 1 19-ounce can Chunky Vegetable Soup. Heat, stirring occasionally. Makes about 3 cups or 2 servings.

Quick Minestrone

Try this with Onion Sandwich Bread or rye crackers for a hearty lunch.

4-5 cups leftover beef or vegetable soup or stew
1 1-pound can tomatoes, chopped
1 cup water or beef or vegetable broth
1 cup shredded cabbage
½ cup elbow macaroni or broken spaghetti*
¼ teaspoon each basil, oregano, and thyme, or to taste
1 1-pound can cannellini, red kidney, or navy beans, drained

Remove and discard any potatoes from leftover soup or stew. Add remaining ingredients, except beans, and simmer 15–20 minutes or until macaroni is tender. Add beans; reheat. Adjust seasonings.

*If you have leftover macaroni or spaghetti on hand, rinse well to remove any starch; drain, and add to soup along with the beans after 10–15 minutes or as soon as the cabbage is cooked.

Hearty Vegetable Medley

The visual impact of this stew will knock you out!

1 small pumpkin
1 red pepper
1 bunch scallions, coarsely chopped
6 small ears corn, cut in thirds or 2 cups kernels*
2 tablespoons oil
2 cloves garlic, minced
2 teaspoons tamari or soy sauce
¼ teaspoon cayenne powder
½ teaspoon salt (optional)

Bake the pumpkin until just tender, about 40–50 minutes in a 350° oven. Let cool until cool enough to handle; peel and cut into 1-inch cubes.

In a large frying pan, sauté the garlic, red pepper, and scallions for 2–3 minutes. Add all remaining ingredients, including pumpkin; cover and steam until corn is cooked, about 5 minutes. Serve as is or over pasta or grain.

*If making this to send off in a thermos, use the corn kernels.

Red Cabbage Soup

For cabbage lovers . . . this soup is almost a stew.

> *1 red or yellow onion, coarsely chopped*
> *2 tablespoons oil*
> *3 cloves garlic, minced*
> *1 small head red cabbage, shredded*
> *3-4 tomatoes or 1 1-pound can tomatoes, peeled and chopped*
> *Salt and pepper to taste*

Sauté onions in oil 5 minutes. Add garlic and cabbage and sauté 5 minutes longer. Add remaining ingredients and as much water as you would like to make a thick soup. Simmer until tender, about 20 minutes. Good with dark bread.

Vegetable Bean Soup

Make a double batch of this nutritious soup. It freezes well which makes it a good choice to have on hand for brown bag lunches.

> *½ pound dry navy beans*
> *1 tablespoon oil*
> *2 cups sliced onions*
> *1 cup diced celery*
> *½ cup diced carrots*
> *1 large clove garlic, minced*
> *1 1-pound can tomatoes*
> *1 teaspoon salt*
> *2 cups diced unpeeled zucchini*
> *½ tablespoon dried basil*
> *½ tablespoon dried parsley*
> *½ teaspoon oregano*

Wash beans; cover with cold water and soak 8 hours or overnight. (Or, simmer 2 minutes; remove from heat, cover, and let stand 1 hour.) Do not drain.

In large pan, heat oil over medium heat. Add onions, celery, carrots, and garlic; cook 5 minutes or until onion is soft. Drain tomatoes, reserving liquid; chop coarsely and add to vegetables. Continue cooking another 3 minutes. Add beans with their liquid and tomato liquid plus enough water to total about 2 quarts of soup. Add salt. Bring to boil; simmer 1½ hours.

Mash some of the beans if a thicker texture is desired; stir in zucchini and remaining seasonings. Cook about 15 minutes or until zucchini is tender. Adjust seasonings.

Chicken Barley Soup

Try this change from the traditional chicken and rice.

³/₄ cup chopped onion
1 clove garlic, minced
3 tablespoons oil
2 chicken legs and thighs (or other favorite chicken parts)
¹/₂-1 cup chopped fresh mushrooms
1¹/₂ cups julienne cut carrots
³/₄ cup diced celery
1 cup barley, rinsed
1 bay leaf
¹/₈ teaspoon each marjoram, parsley, and thyme
Salt and pepper to taste
4-5 cups water or chicken broth

Sauté onion and garlic in oil until golden; add and brown lightly the chicken, mushrooms, and carrots. Add remaining ingredients, using enough water or chicken broth to cover. Simmer 1 hour.

To tote, remove chicken meat from bones; cut into small pieces and return meat to soup. Reheat just before packing into preheated wide mouth vacuum bottle.

Punch up the flavor by adding tomato juice or vegetable cocktail just before serving.

Chilly Tomato Soup

Delightfully refreshing for a hot day. Ripe tomatoes are a must!

1 cup plain yogurt
7 or 8 tomatoes peeled and cut into eighths
Juice and rind of 1 lemon
1 small onion, chopped
1 teaspoon salt (or to taste)
¹/₂ teaspoon dillweed
¹/₄ teaspoon dry mustard
¹/₄ teaspoon thyme
Minced scallions or chives (optional)

Seed tomatoes, if desired. Blend all ingredients in blender until smooth. For serving at home, sprinkle with minced scallions or chives, if desired. Refrigerate until ready to serve.

Package in prechilled thermos.

Cold Cream of Zucchini Soup

Another hot day refresher.

½ cup chopped onion
1 tablespoon oil or butter
1 pound zucchini, sliced
2 cups chicken broth
¼ teaspoon salt
¼ teaspoon oregano
1 cup milk
1 tablespoon flour

In large saucepan, sauté onion in oil or butter until tender but not brown. Add zucchini, broth, salt, and oregano; simmer, covered, until zucchini is just tender. Combine milk and flour in container of electric blender; blend until smooth. Gradually add milk and flour mixture to soup; cook and stir until smooth and slightly thickened. Cool slightly. Pour into container of blender; cover. Blend until smooth. Pour into large covered bowl; chill several hours or overnight before serving or packaging.

To tote: package individual servings in prechilled thermos.

Busy Day Variation: In jar of blender container, combine 1 10¾-ounce can condensed cream of celery soup, 1 cup milk, 1 cup diced cucumber, and salt, pepper, and hot pepper sauce to taste. Blend for 2 minutes. Stir in 1 cup sour cream or yogurt. Chill well. Makes 3½ cups.

Gazpacho

5 ripe tomatoes, peeled and cut in pieces
1 small onion, peeled and cut in pieces
1 clove garlic, minced
4 leaves fresh basil or ½ teaspoon dried basil
2 sprigs fresh parsley or ½ teaspoon dried parsley
1 cup chicken broth
3 tablespoons oil
2 teaspoons vinegar
1 tablespoon lemon juice
⅛ teaspoon paprika
Salt and pepper to taste
For garnish: minced cucumber, red and/or green pepper, and
    sweet onion

Combine all ingredients in blender jar, *except* ingredients for garnish. Cover, blend until smooth, and chill well until ready to serve or pack in prechilled thermos. Sprinkle each serving with some of the garnish or add some to each thermos.

Add punch with a little bit of ground red pepper or bottled hot sauce.

Busy Day Variation: In bowl, combine 1 10¾ ounce can condensed tomato soup, 1 cup water, 1 tablespoon olive oil, 2 tablespoons wine vinegar, and 1 clove garlic, minced. Chill at least 4 hours. Garnish with finely chopped cucumber, green pepper, and onion.

When the Soup is From a Can

This chart of Soup Mates is from the Home Economists of Campbell Kitchens. Use your imagination to create other combinations. (The favorite in our family is Cream of Mushroom + Tomato Bisque + 1 soup can water + 1 soup can milk...served with a grilled cheese sandwich.)

One Soup +	Second Soup +	Liquid = Soup Mate
Bean with Bacon	Beef	1½ soup cans water
Beef	Vegetable Beef	1½ soup cans water
Beef Broth	Tomato	1½ soup cans water
Cream of Celery	Green Pea	1½ soup cans water
Cheddar Cheese	Tomato Bisque	2 soup cans water
Chicken 'n Dumplings	Chicken Vegetable	1½ soup cans water
Chicken Gumbo	Manhattan Clam Chowder	1½ soup cans water
Chicken Gumbo	Chicken Noodle-O's	1½ soup cans water
Chicken Gumbo	Vegetable	1½ soup cans water
Chicken Noodle	Chicken & Stars	1½ soup cans water
Chicken Vegetable	Golden Vegetable Noodle-O's	1½ soup cans water
Chili Beef	Vegetable Beef	1½ soup cans water
Golden Mushroom	Noodles & Ground Beef	1½ soup cans water
Golden Mushroom	Stockpot	1½ soup cans water
Cream of Mushroom	Cream of Shrimp	1 soup can milk + 1 soup can water
Noodles & Ground Beef	Tomato Rice	1½ soup cans water
Onion	Stockpot	1½ soup cans water
Pepper Pot	Vegetable Beef	1½ soup cans water
Split Pea with Ham	Tomato	1 soup can milk + 1 soup can water

Refreshing Apple Soup

4 apples, pared and chopped
½ cup maple syrup or brown sugar
1 teaspoon grated lemon rind
3 cups hot water
½ cup apple juice or white wine
2 tablespoons flour
½ cup milk or cream

Combine apples, maple syrup or sugar, lemon rind, and hot water in saucepan. Simmer apples until tender. Add the apple juice or wine. Combine the flour with 2 tablespoons of water to make a smooth paste and add to the apples. Simmer an additional 5 minutes. Blend on low speed of blender, if desired. Chill well. Add milk or cream just before serving or packaging.

Chilled Strawberries in Wine Soup

2 cups sliced fresh strawberries
⅓ cup honey or sugar
1 cup water
2 teaspoons cornstarch
½ cup white wine or apple juice
1 tablespoon lemon juice
1 teaspoon grated lemon rind

Combine strawberries, honey or sugar, and water in saucepan; simmer until berries are soft. Combine cornstarch with 1 tablespoon water to make a smooth paste and add to the strawberries. Cook and stir until thickened and mixture is clear. Pour into container of electric blender and blend until smooth. Stir in wine or apple juice, lemon, and lemon rind. Chill well before serving or packaging.

It's The Berries! Soup

1 1-pound package frozen blueberries or strawberries
2 cups water
½ cup sugar or maple syrup
3 tablespoons tapioca
Juice and grated rind from 1 large lemon
¼ teaspoon cinnamon

Combine all ingredients in a saucepan. Bring to a boil, stirring constantly. Lower heat and simmer, stirring often, 5 minutes. Refrigerate until well chilled. Serve plain, with tofu whip, whipped sweet or sour cream.

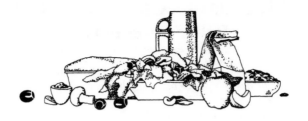

5: Substantial Stuff

Thermos-Cooked Quickies
Pilafs and Pastas
Lunch from Leftovers
'Taters and Toppers to Go

American cuisine reflects its heritage in those foods that we choose to combine into what is loosely categorized as "main dishes." Adventurous cooks not only experiment with ethnic foods, they mix and match seasonings and ingredients to come up with new dishes that bear little resemblance to their original counterparts.

With the exception of our native corn dishes, most American recipes came originally from the Old World with the waves of immigrants who populated this country. As different ethnic groups settled in various parts of the country, we developed regional culinary distinctions that only now are becoming national eating patterns. How? Through the mass marketing and distribution of foods and products that were once available in certain areas of the country only. Now you can buy freshly baked bagels in Texas, hush puppies in Manhattan, and canned refried beans anywhere.

The growing awareness that we average Americans consume too much saturated fats and cholesterol and too little food with adequate starch and fiber has made most of us review our eating habits. We are using a greater variety of complex carbohydrates—such as beans, peas, nuts, seeds, fruits and vegetables, and whole grain products—in the main dishes that we prepare. Interestingly, many of these ingredients return us full circle to the foods of our ancestors; foods that are at their flavorful best when used in some of the old "melting pot" recipes.

THERMOS-COOKED QUICKIES
Italian Pasta-to-Go

Tired of soup and a sandwich? Try this no-cook quickie.

> ⅓ cup small pasta (such as orzo, egg bows, etc.)*
> ¾ cup tomato juice
> ½ cup teaspoon Italian seasoning
> ¼ teaspoon salt
> ⅓ - ½ cup grated firm type cheese

Place pasta in 10-ounce wide mouth thermos. Bring tomato juice and seasonings to a rapid boil; pour over pasta in thermos. Top with cheese. Cap tightly and let stand 1 hour or longer.

*Or use quick cooking vermicelli broken into one-inch lengths. (The brand we used was Skinner/San Giorgio which worked very well.)

Chicken and Bulgur-to-Go

Bulgur has all the quick cooking advantages of processed products but offers the bonus of extra nutrients.

> ½ cup bulgur
> ¼ cup minced cooked chicken
> ¼ cup minced zucchini or cucumber
> 2 tablespoons minced red pepper
> ⅔ cup water
> 2 teaspoons Worcestershire sauce
> ¼ teaspoon basil

Mix bulgur, chicken, zucchini, and red pepper in a 10-ounce wide-mouth thermos. Combine remaining ingredients in a small saucepan and bring to boil. Pour over bulgur mixture; cap, shake well, and let stand one-half hour or longer.

Sweet and Sour Bulgur-to-Go

These ingredients combine well with bulgur's naturally nutty flavor.

> ½ cup bulgur
> 2 tablespoons each: minced apple
>   minced onion
>   red or green cabbage
> ⅔ cup apple juice
> ¼ teaspoon dry mustard
> ¼ teaspoon salt
> 1 teaspoon lemon juice
> 1 teaspoon honey

Mix bulgur, apples, and vegetables in a 10-ounce wide-mouth thermos. In small saucepan, bring apple juice to a boil; stir in remaining ingredients. Pour over bulgur mixture; cap tightly, shake well, and let stand one-half hour or longer.

Travelin' Tetrazzini

⅓ cup vermicelli or very thin spaghetti, regular or quick
  cooking, broken into 1-inch lengths
¾ cup rich chicken broth
1 tablespoon Duxelles, page 125 (optional)
2 tablespoons minced cooked chicken or turkey (optional)
¼ cup grated Parmesan or Romano or ⅓ cup grated Cheddar
  cheese

Preheat 10-ounce wide mouth thermos by filling with boiling water and allowing to stand while preparing remaining ingredients. Drain thermos; place uncooked spaghetti in thermos. Bring chicken broth and Duxelles and chicken, if used, to a full boil. Pour over spaghetti in thermos. Top with cheese. Cap tightly and let stand one hour or longer.

Add punch by substituting 1 or 2 tablespoons of white wine for part of the chicken broth, if desired.

Crunchy Summertime Spaghetti

This unusual recipe is delicious warm, at room temperature or well chilled for a hot day. You could also divide the ingredients between two or three wide mouth thermos bottles and make it as in the recipe above.

1 cup thin or quick cooking spaghetti, broken into 2-3-inch
  lengths
1 can Tomato Garden Soup
1 cup water
1 fresh tomato, peeled and diced
½ teaspoon Italian seasoning

Combine soup, water, tomato, and seasoning in a medium-size saucepan. Bring to a boil and stir in spaghetti so that all pieces are covered by liquid. Cover tightly, remove from heat and let stand 30 minutes. Serve, package for toting, or chill in refrigerator.

To tote, package in prewarmed wide mouth thermos for serving warm or chill several hours or overnight and package in prechilled wide mouth thermos for serving cold. Tuck a separate small package or container of grated cheese into the lunch box if you'd like.

Barbecued Beef

Package this in small containers and freeze for quick reheatable lunches that you can take with a salad or rice, or for stuffing into pita bread.

    2 pounds stew beef, cut in ½-inch pieces
    2 tablespoons butter or margarine
    3 large onions, chopped
    2 cloves garlic, crushed
    ½ cup cider vinegar
    ¼ cup water
    1 tablespoon brown sugar
    2 tablespoons Worcestershire sauce
    ½ cup catsup
    1 teaspoon salt
    2 teaspoons dry mustard

Preheat oven to 325°. Brown meat in butter or margarine. Add remaining ingredients. Turn into covered 2-quart baking dish; bake 2 hours.

Variation: Add 2 cups cooked peas 20 minutes before end of cooking time. Serve over noodles.

Barely Beef Chili

Not too spicy and—consistent with good nutrition practice—this recipe is light on the meat. It also freezes well which makes it a good candidate for your quick lunch freezer shelf.

    ½ pound lean ground beef
    1 cup sliced onion
    1 clove garlic, crushed
    1 green pepper, chopped
    1 28-ounce can tomatoes, broken up
    1 teaspoon salt
    1 bay leaf, crushed
    1 tablespoon chili powder
    1 16-ounce can kidney beans, drained
    ½ cup water or dry red wine

Brown beef and onion in large non-stick frying pan or dutch oven. Add green pepper and garlic; cook and stir until beef is cooked and vegetables are tender. Add tomatoes, salt, bay leaf, and chili powder. Cover and simmer 2 hours. Add the kidney beans and water or wine. Reheat.

Busy Day Variation: In small saucepan in melted butter over medium heat, cook ½ cup diced green pepper until tender. Add 1 19½-ounce can Chunky Chili Beef Soup and ½ cup cooked whole kernel corn. Heat, stirring occasionally. Makes 2 servings.

Lime Chicken

Flavorful, tender chicken that is good hot, warm, or cold. Carry it in your "brown bag" along with a green salad for a low calorie lunch.

6 chicken breast halves or 8 legs, skins removed, if desired
Juice and grated rind of 2 limes
½ cup vegetable oil
½ teaspoon each: salt, paprika, and Tabasco sauce

Place chicken in plastic bag. Combine remaining ingredients; pour over chicken. Close bag tightly; marinate chicken in refrigerator for several hours or overnight, turning occasionally.

Preheat oven to 375°. Place chicken, flesh side down, in shallow baking pan; pour marinade over. Bake, uncovered, 40–50 minutes.

Variation: Substitute ½ cup white wine for the lime juice and rind. Add 1 minced clove garlic, 1 grated small onion and substitute ¼ teaspoon *each* thyme, rosemary, and marjoram for the Tabasco sauce.

Sleeping Chicken

Put this in the oven the night before for lunch the next day or in the morning for a meal that will be ready when you return from work.

3 pounds chicken breasts, skins removed
2 carrots, scrubbed and sliced
2 turnips, pared and cubed
2 celery stalks, sliced
1 onion, sliced
3 cloves garlic, minced
2 cups chicken broth
1 cup beer

Preheat oven to 225°. Combine ingredients in a dutch oven or bean pot. Cover and bake 8–12 hours. Boil the "sauce" down to thicken, if desired. Good served with whole-wheat noodles.

Paella

Bone your own chicken for this recipe and you'll have all those bones to make a pot of rich chicken soup stock.

1 pound boneless chicken, cut into 1-inch cubes
1 small onion, chopped
2 cloves garlic, minced
2 tablespoons salad oil
1½ cups canned or homemade chicken broth
⅔ cup raw regular or converted rice
½ cup chopped canned tomatoes
½ cup chopped green pepper
2 tablespoons chopped pimiento
¼ teaspoon saffron
Salt and pepper to taste

In skillet, brown chicken, onion, and garlic lightly in oil. Add remaining ingredients; cook, covered, over low heat for about 30 minutes or until liquid is absorbed. Stir occasionally. Makes 4 servings.

To tote, reheat and package in preheated wide mouth thermos.

Rice and Vegetable Pie

Not totable but great for Saturday lunch when you have leftover rice.

½ cup chopped onion
2 tablespoons butter or margarine
2 cups cooked rice
¼ teaspoon marjoram
1 slightly beaten egg
¼ cup shredded Cheddar cheese
Salt and pepper to taste
1 small zucchini, halved lengthwise and thinly sliced
1 small tomato, peeled, chopped, and drained
½ cup milk
2 eggs
¼ teaspoon salt
¼ teaspoon marjoram
¾ cup Cheddar cheese

Preheat oven to 350°. Sauté onion in butter or margarine until tender. Remove 1 tablespoon of the onion and combine with rice, marjoram, egg, ¼ cup cheese, and salt and pepper. Press into bottom and sides of a lightly greased 9-inch pie pan. Sprinkle with zucchini, tomato, and remaining sautéed onion. Beat together milk, 2 eggs, salt, and marjoram; pour over vegetables; sprinkle with the ¾ cup cheese. Bake 45 minutes or until set. Let stand 5 minutes before cutting.

Spanish Rice

An old favorite in our home and a good thermos choice—the flavors blend and carry well.

2 tablespoons oil
2 tablespoons tamari or soy sauce (optional)
1 medium onion, chopped
1 red or green pepper, chopped
1 cup brown rice
$1/2$ teaspoon chili powder
$1/4$ teaspoon thyme
$1/8$–$1/4$ teaspoon cayenne pepper
$1/2$ cup black olives, sliced
2–3 tomatoes, peeled and sliced
2 cups boiling water
Salt and pepper to taste
Parmesan cheese (optional)

Heat oil and tamari sauce in large frying pan. Sauté the onion and pepper in the oil until golden. Stir in rice and sauté a minute longer, stirring so that all grains are coated with oil. Add remaining ingredients. Slowly pour in water. Cover and simmer 40–50 minutes. Sprinkle with Parmesan cheese, if desired.

To tote, reheat if necessary and package in wide mouth thermos.

Crunchy Kasha

Kasha is a readily available, quick cooking, nutritious grain—perfect for a winter day.

1 tablespoon oil
1 medium onion, chopped
1 cup kasha
$1/2$ cup sunflower seeds
1 cup cooked pumpkin cubes or sliced raw zucchini
$2 1/2$ cups vegetable broth

Sauté onions in the oil until golden; add kasha and stir until lightly toasted. Add remaining ingredients, cover, and simmer about 20 minutes.

To tote, package in wide mouth thermos.

Zucchini and Tomato Frittata

Any combination of vegetables to equal approximately 3 cups can re-place the zucchini.

3 medium zucchini, halved lengthwise and thinly sliced
1 large onion or 2 leeks, thinly sliced
2 cloves garlic, minced
2 tomatoes, peeled and chopped
¼ cup sunflower, corn, or olive oil
6 eggs, lightly beaten
½ teaspoon Italian seasoning
¼ teaspoon salt
¼ teaspoon freshly ground pepper
⅔ cup grated Romano or Parmesan cheese

Preheat oven to 375°. Sauté all vegetables in oil 5 minutes on high heat, stirring occasionally. Spoon into a greased 8 × 11 × 2-inch baking dish (or roughly equivalent size). Pour beaten eggs over; sprinkle with cheese and seasonings. Bake 30 minutes.

LEFTOVERS THAT ADD UP TO LUNCH

Lunch time is a good time to use up the bits and pieces that have been accumulating in the refrigerator. Whether eaten at home, carried off in a brown bag, or prepared to stash in the freezer for a quick reheatable lunch on a busy day, madeover leftovers can provide some interesting alternatives to the routine sandwich.

Clean Out The Fridge Quiche

This is almost as fast as cleaning out the fridge and infinitely more pleasing to the palate.

1 9- or 10-inch unbaked pastry shell
2 cups mixed cooked vegetables and/or grains
1 onion, minced
3 eggs
1 cup vegetable broth or tomato juice
1 cup grated Cheddar or Swiss cheese
½ teaspoon salt
1 teaspoon marjoram, rosemary, or herb of your choice
1 teaspoon prepared mustard

Preheat oven to 375°. Mix all ingredients, *except* pastry shell, together with a whisk or wooden spoon. Pour into a 9- or 10-inch unbaked pieshell. Bake 30 minutes.

Tuna Tomato Tart

Good hot or cold, this makes a good traveler.

Pastry for 9-inch pie crust
1 cup chopped onion
2 cloves garlic, minced
¼ cup oil
1 7-ounce can tuna, drained and flaked
1½ cups peeled, chopped tomatoes (fresh or canned)
½ cup olives, minced
3 eggs, slightly beaten
½ cup milk or water or tomato juice
½ cup Parmesan cheese
2 teaspoons Italian seasoning
1 teaspoon salt (optional)

Preheat oven to 400°. Use prepared pastry to line 8-inch square pan, turning up sides about 1-inch. Sauté onion and garlic in oil until tender. Stir in remaining ingredients. Pour into pie crust lined pan. Bake ½ hour.

To tote, cut cold leftover tart into squares to fit plastic sandwich boxes.

Noodle Omelet

Have you ever wondered what to do with a cup of leftover noodles?

4 eggs, lightly beaten
¾ - 1 cup leftover cooked noodles or macaroni and cheese
½ teaspoon salt
1 - 2 tablespoons margarine or butter
2 tablespoons grated Romano cheese (optional)
Freshly ground pepper to taste

In medium-size frying pan, heat margarine over medium heat. Combine remaining ingredients until well blended. When margarine is melted, pour in egg mixture and cook just until bottom and sides are set. Remove from heat. Loosen omelet with a spatula; flip over one side, folding the omelet in half; cover pan and let stand for a few minutes until the center of the omelet is "set." Slip out onto serving plate. Serves 2.

Nutty Noodle Loaf

This one is good for those days when the fridge is loaded with a variety of leftovers.

1 small onion, minced
½ cup finely chopped almonds or walnuts
2 tablespoons oil
2 cups leftover cooked noodles
2 cups leftover cooked mixed vegetables
2 packages frozen mustard greens or spinach, thawed and well drained
3 eggs, lightly beaten
1 cup cottage cheese or crumbled tofu
¾ cup vegetable stock or tomato juice

Preheat oven to 350°. Sauté onion and nuts until golden. Combine with all remaining ingredients. Grease a 9 × 5 × 3-inch loaf pan; dust pan with cornstarch or arrowroot. Pack mixture into pan, smoothing out top. Bake 35–45 minutes. Turn out of pan and slice; serve plain or with tomato sauce.

Pizza Pronto

No waiting for the dough to rise; just mix and bake!

½ cup whole-wheat flour
½ cup unbleached all-purpose flour
½ teaspoon baking powder
⅛ teaspoon salt
¼ cup water
2 tablespoons olive, corn, or sunflower oil
Cornmeal
½ cup tomato or pizza sauce
1 small onion, sliced
4 mushrooms, sliced (optional)
½ teaspoon oregano
¾ cup grated Cheddar or mozzarella cheese

Preheat oven to 425°. Combine first six ingredients and knead several times until smooth. Shape dough into a ball; roll out into a 10–12-inch circle. Place on a greased cookie sheet or pizza pan which has been sprinkled with cornmeal. Pinch outer edges as when shaping a pie crust.

Spread sauce on crust, then layer remaining ingredients. Sprinkle with additional 1–2 teaspoons of oil, if desired. Bake 20–25 minutes.

BLT Rice

This is especially fast and easy if you have "planned ahead" leftover cooked bacon in the refrigerator.

¼ pound bacon, cooked and crumbled into pieces
1 large onion, chopped
2 tablespoons oil (or bacon fat)
3 cups cold leftover cooked rice
1 tablespoon white wine
2 tablespoons water
¼ head lettuce, shredded
1 large tomato, peeled and chopped
2 tablespoons tamari or soy sauce

If not using leftover bacon: cook bacon until crisp, set aside to drain on paper towels while cooking onions. Sauté onion in oil or bacon fat. Add wine and water. Pile rice on top and steam, covered, 1 minute. Stir in all remaining ingredients and heat.

To tote, spoon into preheated wide mouth vacuum bottle. Add a small container of grated cheese, if desired.

Soup Plus Makes A Hot Meal

A pattern recipe from the Campbell Soup people that can be the basis for a wide variety of quick lunches.

½ cup cooked meat or poultry, cut in strips
1 tablespoon butter or margarine
1 can any Campbell's Soup
1 soup can milk or water
½ cup cooked vegetables

In saucepan, cook meat in butter until lightly browned. Add remaining ingredients. Heat; stir often. Makes about 2½ cups.

Add punch by sautéing a bit of minced onion with the meat or adding a bit of your favorite dried herb that is compatible with the soup you are using.

To tote, spoon into preheated wide mouth vacuum bottle.

Salad Plus Makes A Cold Meal

Leftover, properly stored, salads can be the basis for a quickly prepared lunch or different side dish the next day. To tote, remember to chill well before packing in a prechilled wide mouth thermos.

To leftover:	Add:
Macaroni Salad	Tuna fish + sweet relish + diced fresh tomato, if desired + additional mayonnaise or yogurt to taste
	Cubed ham or bologna and/or cubed Swiss cheese + chopped green pepper + additional dressing and mustard
	Crumbled, cooked bacon + chopped hard-cooked eggs + creamy onion or Russian dressing and/or mustard
Rice Salad	Ham or cooked, crumbled bacon + diced green pepper + chopped fresh tomato
	Cooked shrimp, cut in pieces + shredded carrot + lemon juice to taste
	Shrimp or crabmeat + additional mayonnaise and chili sauce to thin and season
	Tuna fish or shrimp + celery + French Dressing to thin + ½ teaspoon curry for each 2 cups of salad
Potato Salad	Slivers of cooked roast beef + chopped green pepper or chives + cold, cooked green beans, if desired + Italian Dressing or additional mayonnaise or yogurt to taste
	Diced hard-cooked eggs + slivers of salami + chopped pickles or olives, if desired + mustard
Chicken Salad	Drained mandarin orange sections, seedless grapes, and/or pineapple tidbits + slivered almonds + additional mayonnaise or yogurt as needed to extend salad.
	Cubed ham or crumbled bacon + leftover rice, if desired + additional mayonnaise or yogurt to taste
	Unpared, cubed apples + celery + slivered almonds + additional dressing, heavy cream, or yogurt to thin

Ham Salad	Chopped hard-cooked eggs and/or cubed cheese + additional dressing and mustard
Seafood Salad	Additional celery + cold leftover rice + additional mayonnaise + ½ teaspoon curry or 1 tablespoon chili sauce for each 2 cups of rice
Coleslaw	Diced, unpared red apples + broken walnuts + dark raisins + additional mayonnaise or yogurt to thin
Sauerkraut	Peeled, sliced apples + finely chopped onion + chopped celery + oil and vinegar, if desired

'TATERS WITH TOPPERS TO GO

For a hearty luncheon main dish, try a baked potato with a zestful topping. Popular restaurants feature this favorite on their menus but you can enjoy it at home or away—if your place of employment is one of the many that has a microwave oven for use by its employees.

The Perfect Baked Potato

For each serving, scrub potato, dry well and pierce in several places with a fork to allow steam to escape. Don't wrap the potatoes in foil!

To bake in conventional oven: Place large (8–10-ounce) potatoes directly on oven rack in a 425° oven. Bake 50–60 minutes or until potato feels soft when pierced with a skewer.

To bake in microwave oven: Arrange medium-size (6–8-ounce) potatoes in microwave, leaving 1-inch between them. (For more than 2 potatoes, arrange them in a circle and turn and rearrange them once during the microwaving cycle.) Microwave at High for times shown:

Number of Potatoes:	Minutes at HIGH*
1	4 to 6
2	6 to 8
3	8 to 12
4	12 to 16
5	16 to 20

*Potatoes may still feel firm when done; let stand up to 5 minutes to soften. Allow additional baking time if using large potatoes.

When potatoes are done, use a fork to cut an X in the top and squeeze the potato gently to fluff up the pulp.

Spud Sauces

A check of your refrigerator and pantry will probably turn up a number of toppings that require almost no preparation. Sour cream or yogurt; grated or cubed cheeses like Cheddar, fontina, or Monterey Jack or cheese sauce; leftover ratatouille, chili, or Swedish meatballs; slivers of roast beef with thin slices of onion; undiluted, heated cream of mushroom soup; Cream Cheese Herb or Bacon Salad Dressing—the possibilities are limited only by your imagination and supply of leftovers.

When time allows, try some of these special 'tater topper sauces:

Orange Yogurt Topping

1 tablespoon margarine
1 tablespoon flour
½ cup orange juice
1 tablespoon grated orange rind
1 cup plain yogurt, at room temperature

Melt margarine; stir in flour. Slowly stir in juice and cook until thickened. Remove from heat; stir in rind and yogurt. Spoon over potatoes or steamed vegetables.

Golden Cheese Sauce

1 cup beer (regular, lite, or leftover flat beer)
½ cup water
2 tablespoons cornstarch
¾ cup grated cheese, preferably Cheddar
1 teaspoon prepared mustard, preferably Dijon

Combine all ingredients in saucepan and bring to boil over medium heat, stirring constantly, until thick and smooth.

Mushroom Sauce

¼ pound mushrooms, sliced
1 small onion, minced
2 tablespoons margarine
1 tablespoon flour
1 cup chicken or vegetable broth
1 tablespoon white wine or sherry
⅛ teaspoon salt
Dash nutmeg (optional)

Sauté mushrooms and onion 5 minutes over medium heat. Stir in flour. Gradually stir in broth, wine, and seasonings. Cook several minutes, stirring constantly, until thick and smooth.

Lemony Egg Sauce

1 tablespoon margarine
1 tablespoon flour (or 2 tablespoons for a thick sauce)
1 cup chicken or vegetable broth or milk
¼ teaspoon each: salt and pepper
1 or 2 hard-cooked eggs, chopped
1 teaspoon grated lemon rind
1 teaspoon lemon juice
Dash nutmeg (optional)

Melt margarine in small saucepan. Stir in flour. Gradually stir in broth or milk, salt, and pepper. Cook several minutes, stirring constantly, until thick and smooth. Gently stir in eggs, rind, and juice.

Creamy Italian Sauce

This sauce is equally good over pasta!

½ cup each: minced onion
                minced red or green pepper
                minced celery
3 tablespoons oil, preferably olive oil
1 tablespoon flour
½ cup ricotta cheese
½ cup grated mozzarella cheese
½ cup milk or water
½ teaspoon salt
½ teaspoon oregano

Sauté vegetables in oil until barely tender. Stir in all remaining ingredients. Cook and stir over very low heat until cheese is melted.

Tuna Barbecue Sauce

1 7-ounce can chunk style tuna, drained
1 8-ounce can tomato sauce
½ cup minced onion
¼ cup catsup
¼ cup apple juice
1 tablespoon tamari or soy sauce
¼ teaspoon oregano
¼ teaspoon paprika
2 tablespoons oil

Combine all ingredients in a small saucepan and simmer 10–15 minutes. Stir in tuna. *For a thicker sauce:* stir 2 tablespoons cornstarch *or* arrowroot into a small amount of water. Stir into sauce before adding tuna; cook and stir until clear and thickened.

Wine Sauce

½ cup minced mushrooms
½ cup minced onions
1 tablespooon margarine or oil
1 cup white or red wine
1 bay leaf
½ teaspoon Italian seasoning
¼ teaspoon salt
2 tablespoons cornstarch or arrowroot

Sauté mushrooms and onions in oil for 1 minute over high heat, stirring constantly. Add wine and seasonings; simmer 10 minutes. Remove bay leaf. Stir cornstarch or arrowroot into a small amount of water; stir into sauce. Cook and stir until thickened and smooth.

Pesto for Potatoes

¹/₄ cup chopped fresh basil leaves
¹/₄ cup walnuts, almonds, or pine nuts
¹/₄ cup Romano or Parmesan cheese
2 cloves garlic
¹/₄ cup oil, preferably olive or sunflower oil
¹/₈ teaspoon each: salt and pepper

Place all ingredients in blender; blend until as smooth or chunky as you like it.

Cold Sauce for Potatoes

½ cup mayonnaise or sour cream
½ cup applesauce, preferably unsweetened
1 teaspoon prepared horseradish

Blend ingredients together with a whisk or fork. Serve cold or at room temperature.

To tote 'taters and toppers: Carry scrubbed, pierced potato wrapped in a paper towel ready to pop into microwave. Package topping separately in a small microwave safe container so that you can reheat it, if you desire. To reheat, cover container with plastic wrap to prevent spatters and place in microwave with potatoes for last 1–1½ minutes. Watch carefully so that sauce does not boil over.

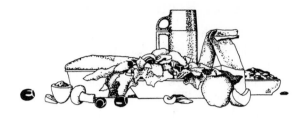

6: Savory Salads and Such

Greens and Grains
Other Veggies and Pastas
Finger Foods and Dips
Gelatin Salads
Fruit Salads
Dressings

It has taken fruits and vegetables a long time to gain prominence in our diets. The Greeks ate dried peas, radishes, cabbages, lettuce, and turnips; the Romans enjoyed cucumbers, asparagus, and leeks as well. But history gives little evidence that vegetables and fruits—as we know them today—played a major role in dietary habits.

Most of our common fruits and vegetables first were brought into cultivation in the Eastern hemisphere. The Indians of the New World developed cultivation of the potato, tomato, corn, and some varieties of squash. But many vegetables and fruits have been available in the wild or under cultivation longer than men have dared—or deigned—to eat them. What better example than the all-American favorite, the tomato, which was commonly regarded as poisonous until the last century! Fortunately, improved methods of handling and shipping now enable us to enjoy foods that either were unknown or were rare treats to our forefathers.

Today, fewer lunch boxes are loaded with pasty white bread or high-sugar/simple carbohydrate convenience foods. The salad—tossed, molded, or marinated vegetables or fruit—is rapidly catching up to the sandwich as a brown bag favorite. Accompanied by whole-grain breads, cheese and small portions of other protein foods, it satisfies the changing American preference for a little "crunch" and "munch"—and better nutrition with fewer calories.

Ever-Ready Salad Bar

Great salads require fresh, clean, crisp greens—a preparation chore that no one wants to face at six in the morning. A small investment in super-sized containers* will provide you with a "salad bar" that will give you the "fixings" for a week of crisp salads. The few nutrients lost from advance preparation will be more than offset by the fact that you will serve salads much more often.

Start by washing vegetables thoroughly. Use plenty of water for leafy greens, washing them in several changes of cool water and lifting them from the water so that soil that settles in the bottom of the pan will not be drained back through the vegetables. Remove bruised, wilted, or tough parts but trim sparingly so that valuable nutrients will not be wasted. (Never use a metal knife implement that could encourage rust to develop on the greens; instead, save a plastic picnic knife for tasks like removing the core from lettuce.) Shake well in a colander or use a salad spinner to remove excess water; then set on a paper towel to complete draining.

Line a large container with several thicknesses of paper towels. Pile greens in lightly (place lettuce in cored side down); cover with another paper towel and the lid. Refrigerate.

Clean carrots, celery, peppers, broccoli, cauliflower, and other vegetables that can add crunch to your lunch. Trim and cut into sticks or florets for grab-and-run finger foods, then store in a plastic bag or container lined with damp paper towel. These will stay fresh for four or five days in the refrigerator, ready "as is" as finger foods, or handy for slicing into smaller pieces for tossed salads.

Keep containers used for storing prepared vegetables scrupulously clean. But avoid using soapy water which could leave a film that would develop a sour odor with time. Wash containers with baking soda and warm water, rinse thoroughly with hot water, and dry well.

* The refrigerator crisper drawer is fine for storing many fruits and vegetables but salad greens are happier if you keep a tight lid on humidity. The container that I have used for more years than I can remember is the Freezette® 9½ quart #139 Flat container which measures approximately 14 × 10 × 5 inches. [A Snap-Lok (#339) is also available but I prefer the easier access of the standard cover.] The Tupperware Easy Crisp® container is marvelous for celery, carrot sticks and other finger foods because it has a special grid on the bottom that stores vegetables above the moisture.

Chef's Salad

6 cups torn salad greens: leaf or head lettuce, endive, escarole
romaine
½ cup sliced celery
3 scallions, snipped
1 medium tomato, cut in wedges
¼-inch slice boiled ham (about 4-ounces), cut in thin strips
2 1-ounce slices Swiss cheese
2 hard-cooked eggs, cut in quarters

Toss vegetables together lightly; arrange remaining ingredients on top. Serve with salad dressing of choice. Makes 3–4 servings.

Vary this basic recipe by substituting chunks of solid white tuna or leftover cooked chicken, or slivers of salami or bologna for the ham. Try other favorite cheeses—Cheddar, Monterey Jack, Gorgonzola—or cubes of well-drained tofu.

Add crunch by tossing in a few crisp florets of raw broccoli or cauliflower or tender asparagus tips. Garnish with a few cooked chick peas, raw sprouts, or seasoned croutons just before tossing.

To tote: Toss vegetables together and pile each serving in a plastic container with a leak-proof cover (a 1¼-quart size would be about right). Divide remaining ingredients between servings and place in plastic sandwich bags on top of salads. Cover tightly and place in insulated lunch bag. (Don't forget a separate small container of salad dressing.)

Mandarin Special

A refreshing main dish salad for a hot day.

6 cups torn lettuce or assorted salad greens
1 cup tangerine sections or 1 11-ounce can Mandarin orange
segments, well-drained
½ cup sliced green pepper
½ cup diced celery
1 cup diced cooked chicken

Chill salad greens. Combine remaining ingredients and chill separately. When ready to serve, combine and toss together lightly with dressing of your choice (or regular or tofu mayonnaise thinned with a bit of orange juice and flavored with grated orange rind).

To tote, package salad greens in large container. Combine remaining ingredients, wrap loosely in plastic wrap or foil and set on top of salad greens. Package salad dressing in separate small container. Remove plastic or foil wrap at serving time; add salad dressing.

Chunky Chicken Waldorf

This combines two all-time favorite salads with zesty results.

2 cups cooked chicken or turkey, in large chunks
½ cup sliced celery
1 teaspoon grated onion
1 cup diced unpared apple
¼ cup yogurt
¼ cup mayonnaise
1 tablespoon lemon juice or vinegar
Salt and pepper to taste

Combine chicken, celery, onion, apple. In separate small bowl, mix yogurt with mayonnaise, lemon juice or vinegar, and salt and pepper; toss with chicken mixture. Refrigerate.

To tote, package in prechilled wide mouth thermos jars.

Add crunch by stirring in ¼–½ cup chopped walnuts or slivered almonds.

Spinach Salad with Spicy Mushrooms

Try this alternative to the customary bacon dressing.

½ pound fresh mushrooms, thickly sliced
1 medium-size sweet onion, thinly sliced
⅓ cup salad oil
¼ cup cider or wine vinegar
1–2 drops hot pepper sauce
1 tablespoon fresh minced parsley or 1 teaspoon dried parsley
Salt and pepper to taste
½ pound fresh spinach

Combine mushrooms and onions in bowl; add remaining ingredients and mix gently. Cover and let stand at room temperature for 2 hours or refrigerate overnight.

Meanwhile, wash and dry spinach; chill well. When ready to serve or prepare salad for packaging, tear spinach into salad bowl or serving size covered container, discarding coarse stems. Toss with marinated mushroom dressing just before serving. Makes enough for two luncheon salads or four small side salads.

To tote, package spinach in prechilled large covered container and marinated mushroom dressing in small separate container.

Stuffed Chard-to-Go

These are traditionally eaten at room temperature.

1 large bunch Swiss chard
¾ cup minced onions
2 or 3 cloves garlic, minced
2 tablespoons oil
½ cup fresh parsley or chives, minced
2 cups cooked rice
½ teaspoon salt
1–3 tablespoons fresh mint, minced (optional)
2 tablespoons tahini (optional)

Clean Swiss chard and remove any very thick ribs. Cover with boiling water and let stand while preparing filling. Sauté onions and garlic in oil until tender; mix in remaining ingredients. Drain Swiss chard well and pat dry with paper towel if necessary. Spoon a tablespoon of filling in the center of each leaf and fold up envelope fashion. Place in a heavy saucepan. Cover with 1 cup boiling water and simmer 30 minutes. Cool, drain off water and refrigerate overnight (or several days if desired), and serve at room temperature. Good with cherry tomatoes or olives and cubes of feta cheese. Makes 2–3 dozen.

Add crunch by adding ¼ cup pine nuts to the filling.

Lunchpail Rice Special

A savory salad that lends itself to variation.

1½ cups cold, cooked rice
2 tomatoes, peeled, coarsely chopped, drained of excess juice
½ red pepper, finely chopped
2 tablespoons oil
1 tablespoon vinegar
1 teaspoon prepared mustard
1 teaspoon tamari or salt and pepper to taste
¼ cup roasted sunflower seeds
1 cup shredded lettuce

Combine all ingredients well. Serve immediately or chill until time to package in 2 10-ounce insulated jars.

Variation: Substitute ½ cup diced ham or shrimp for ½ cup of the lettuce.

Rice and Egg Salad

This is good cold or at room temperature.

2 cups cooked rice (cooled to room temperature)
2 hardcooked eggs, minced
2 stalks celery, minced
1 small onion, minced
¼ cup mayonnaise
2 tablespoons oil
1 tablespoon vinegar, preferably white wine vinegar
½ teaspoon salt
1 tablespoon prepared mustard or tahini

Mix all ingredients together and chill, if desired. Good stuffed into to-matoes (especially cherry tomatoes) or spread on romaine and rolled up jellyroll fashion for eating as a breadless sandwich.

Tabbouleh

Or, Tabuli, or, Tabooli. However you spell it, this nutritious salad is great to have on hand in the refrigerator. (It keeps well for a week.)

¾ cup bulgur (cracked wheat)
1 large tomato, peeled and diced
1 medium onion, chopped
¼ cup minced fresh parsley
¼ cup minced fresh mint
6 tablespoons salad or olive oil
3 tablespoons lemon juice
1 teaspoon salt
Pepper to taste

Pour boiling water over bulgur in medium-size bowl. Cover and let stand 30 minutes or until bulgur is soft. Drain well. Add tomato, onion, parsley, and mint; mix lightly but well. Combine oil and lemon juice with salt and pepper in small jar; cover and shake well to blend. Pour over bulgur and vegetables; mix well. Chill, covered, several hours or overnight. Serve on salad greens, if desired.

Variation: Omit the tomato from the salad and use the salad to stuff tomatoes.

Deliciously Different Bulgur

Make this the night before so that all the seasonings have a chance to "get acquainted."

>   *1½ cups bulgur*
>   *1½ cups boiling water*
>   *2 medium onions, chopped*
>   *3 tablespoons margarine or oil*
>   *1 tablespoon flour*
>   *1 cup favorite soup stock*
>   *1 tablespoon wine or cider vinegar*
>   *1 tablespoon prepared mustard*
>   *½ teaspoon salt*
>   *2 small zucchini, chopped*
>   *1 cup cooked chickpeas (optional)*

Pour boiling water over bulgur and let stand 20–30 minutes. Meanwhile, prepare "dressing." Sauté onion in margarine or oil until translucent. Stir in flour. Slowly stir in remaining ingredients, *except zucchini and chickpeas.* Cook and stir 2 minutes. Pour over bulgur while hot. Cover and refrigerate at least one hour. Stir in zucchini and chickpeas before serving or packaging.

To tote, package in prechilled wide mouth thermos jar. Good with a separate green salad and fresh fruit for dessert.

Tangy Greek Salad

Serve as a side dish or with leftover cooked pasta or cubes of firm tofu.

>   *4 ounces feta or goat cheese, crumbled or diced*
>   *1 pint basket cherry tomatoes, halved*
>   *1 red onion, sliced and separated into rings*
>   *½ green pepper, slivered*
>   *2 small zucchini, halved lengthwise and sliced*
>   *1 8-ounce can pitted black olives, drained and halved*
>   *¼ cup oil, preferably olive oil*
>   *2 tablespoons wine vinegar*
>   *⅛ teaspoon salt*
>   *½ teaspoon parsley*
>   *½ teaspoon oregano or basil*

Combine vegetables in a bowl or large jar. Shake oil, vinegar, and seasonings in a small jar to blend. Pour over salad. Marinate for at least 30 minutes. Will keep 5 days, covered, in refrigerator.

Number One Noodle Salad

A good traveler but check the Onion Lover's Tip on page 106!

8 ounces thin noodles, preferably whole-grain, cooked
3 tablespoons oil
1 tablespoon vinegar, preferably rice
1 tablespoon maple syrup or frozen apple juice concentrate
2 tablespoons tamari or soy sauce
1 bunch scallions, sliced in ½-inch pieces
1 clove garlic, minced

In small bowl or covered jar, mix all ingredients, *except* noodles, until well combined. Pour over noodles. Eat immediately or refrigerate until time to package.

Pasta and Tofu Salad

8 ounces uncooked whole-wheat noodles or macaroni
8 ounces firm tofu
1 tablespoon tamari sauce
1 tablespoon vinegar
1 tablespoon oil
1 bunch scallions, sliced
½ red pepper or carrot, slivered

Cook noodles or macaroni according to package directions; drain well. Drain tofu well and cut into ¼–½-inch cubes. Mix all ingredients together well. Chill before serving or packaging. Serve as is or with your choice of dressing.

Deli Style Macaroni Salad

½ pound macaroni, cooked and drained
2 vegetable broth cubes dissolved in ¼ cup hot water
¾ cup plain yogurt or sour cream
1 cup mayonnaise
½ teaspoon salt
¼ teaspoon freshly grated black pepper
½ cup minced red onion
½ cup minced green pepper
¼ cup pickle relish
1 teaspoon dillweed

Combine ¼ cup of the yogurt with the dissolved broth cubes and water; pour over warm cooked macaroni. Mix all remaining ingredients together; pour over macaroni; mix well. Chill before serving.

Macaroni and Tuna Salad

Pickled beets and onions with cottage cheese are a marvelous complement to this salad.

1 cup uncooked elbow macaroni
1 7-ounce can tuna
1 tablespoon grated onion
2 tablespoons sweet pickle relish
1 tablespoon minced parsley
¾ cup egg or tofu mayonnaise
½ teaspoon salt
¼ teaspoon pepper

Cook, drain, and cool macaroni. Mix in remaining ingredients. Chill.

New Potato Salad

Here is one potato salad you can serve warm for dinner one night and chilled for lunch the next day.

½ pound new potatoes
½ teaspoon salt
½ cup mayonnaise
Grated rind and juice from ½ lemon or lime
2 tablespoons fresh minced chives, parsley, or dill
Freshly grated pepper

Scrub potatoes well; pare a thin strip of skin from the middle. In saucepan, cover with water. Bring to a boil; cover and simmer until tender, about 15–20 minutes. Drain well. Cut potatoes in half, if desired. Mix remaining ingredients and spoon over potatoes; toss lightly to mix.

Sweet or White Potato Salad

2 pounds white or sweet potatoes
3 stalks celery, thinly sliced
1 medium carrot, thinly sliced
⅓ cup oil
¼ cup apple cider vinegar
1 tablespoon chopped parsley
2 scallions, minced
2 teaspoons prepared mustard
1 teaspoon salt

Steam potatoes until tender; peel and cube while still warm. Toss potatoes with celery and carrots. Combine remaining ingredients in a screw top jar and shake until well blended. Pour over vegetables and toss lightly. Refrigerate for at least one hour or overnight.

Quick Coleslaw

A "must" for picnics or cold suppers, coleslaw also makes a nice addition to the brown bag.

1 medium head cabbage, shredded
1 cup egg or tofu mayonnaise
2 tablespoons mustard, preferably Dijon
2 tablespoons white wine vinegar or apple cider vinegar
½ cup minced onion
½ cup coarsely shredded carrot (optional)

Toss all ingredients together. Chill for at least 1 hour.

Add punch by doubling the amount of mustard used or by adding a sprinkling of celery seed.

Vary the flavor by substituting sour cream for half of the mayonnaise.

Sunshine Salad

1½ cup grated carrots
½ cup raisins
½ cup chopped nuts
Mayonnaise

Combine carrots, raisins, and nuts with enough mayonnaise to moisten; toss lightly. Chill.

Vary the flavor by adding chopped celery, apples, or well drained crushed pineapple.

Speedy Bean Salad

1 15- or 20-ounce can canneloni beans
1 red onion, chopped
1 pint cherry tomatoes, halved or 1 red pepper, chopped
1 medium-size zucchini or cucumber, chopped
¼ cup oil
2 tablespoons vinegar
Juice and grated rind from ½ lime or lemon
½ cup minced chives or scallions
¼ cup yogurt (optional)

Mix beans and vegetables in a bowl or jar. Shake remaining ingredients together until smooth; pour over vegetables. Chill 1 hour. Keeps 5 days.

Tip for onion lovers: Pack a few sprigs of fresh parsley in your lunch box. Just chew on them to freshen your breath after you have indulged in your favorite "flavor enhancer."

Bountiful Bean Salad

For the very best in bean salads, make this with freshly cooked beans whenever you have time.

1 ⅓ cups cider vinegar or wine vinegar
⅔ cup vegetable oil
¾ cup sugar
2 teaspoons salt (or to taste)
1 teaspoon pepper
1 large red or yellow onion, chopped
1 small green pepper, chopped (optional)
1 cup chopped celery
1 16-ounce can cut green beans or 2 cups cooked fresh green
  beans
1 16-ounce can yellow wax beans or 2 cups cooked fresh wax
  beans
1 16-ounce can red kidney beans or 2 cups cooked dry kidney
  beans
1 16-ounce can chick peas (garbanzos) or 2 cups cooked dry
  chick peas

Drain all beans thoroughly and mix. Heat first five ingredients until sugar is dissolved. Pour sauce over beans; gently stir in remaining ingredients. Pour into glass jars or containers with tight lids or screw tops and store in refrigerator. Let stand at least overnight in refrigerator before serving. Keeps several weeks in refrigerator.

Serve as relish or salad with almost anything.

Punch up the flavor of tossed green salad with the addition of a few spoonfuls of well drained Bean Salad.

Chick Peas Remoulade

Try this delightful salad stuffed into a fresh, ripe tomato or served on a bed of shredded lettuce. Good as an appetizer, too.

1 20-ounce can chick peas, drained
½ cup celery, finely diced
¼ cup mayonnaise
2 tablespoons sweet pickle relish
2 tablespoons chili sauce
2 teaspoons Worcestershire sauce

Combine ingredients well; chill.

FINGER FOODS AND DIPS
Ham and Cheese Roll-ups

An easy finger food that goes well with a side salad—a popular combination for dieters.

> *1 8-ounce package of light cream cheese, at room temperature*
> *1 tablespoon milk or cream*
> *2 teaspoons prepared horseradish or 1 tablespoon minced scallions*
> *½ teaspoon prepared mustard (optional)*
> *4-5 slices thinly sliced boiled ham*

Beat cream cheese with milk or cream until light and fluffy; stir in horseradish or scallions and mustard. Spread on slices of ham. Roll up ham jelly-roll fashion, starting at narrow end. Wrap in foil or plastic wrap and chill several hours or overnight.

Add punch to this recipe by substituting yogurt cheese, page 52, for cream cheese.

To tote, package as is in an insulated container or bag or unwrap and cut into thick slices and arrange slices in a prechilled thermos jar.

Devilish Chicken Fingers with Honey Dip

Be as devilish as you dare by using hot mustard—or stirring in a little extra dry mustard.

> *2-3 pounds favorite chicken parts or 1-1½ pounds boneless chicken breasts*
> *½ cup melted butter or margarine*
> *2 tablespoons flour*
> *2 tablespoons prepared mustard*
> *½ cup cornflake crumbs*
> *½ cup yellow cornmeal*
> *1 teaspoon salt*
> *¼ teaspoon paprika*

Preheat oven to 350°. Remove skin from chicken parts and bone chicken breasts if necessary. Separate legs from thighs, if necessary, and cut each boneless half breast in half lengthwise. Blend flour and mustard into melted butter until smooth. Dip chicken pieces in butter mixture and coat well with combined crumbs and seasonings. Place on shallow foil-lined pan and drizzle with any remaining butter mixture. Bake 35–40 minutes or until tender. Refrigerate.

To tote: Package chicken in prechilled wide-mouth thermos; add a separate container of honey for dipping.

Big and Little Dippers

Finger foods and dips make easy, totable lunches and they're fun. Most dips stay fresh for several days in the refrigerator—ready to go with some crunchy vegetables, fruit, or other "go-withs." Here are some suggestions for good dippers and recipes for dips to accompany them.

Raw Vegetables: Asparagus tips, broccoli or cauliflower buds, carrot and celery sticks, cucumber or zucchini sticks, green pepper chunks, radishes, scallions, cherry tomatoes or tomato wedges.

Raw Fruit: Apple or pear slices (dipped in lemon juice to prevent darkening or carried whole and cut up at lunchtime), cantaloupe wedges, mandarin oranges (canned), melon balls, pineapple sticks, seedless grapes, strawberries.

Seafood and Poultry: Bite-size chunks of tuna, crab-meat, lobster tail, or leftover cold, cooked fish fillets or scallops, whole shrimp; Devilish Chicken Fingers (page 108), legs or bite-size chunks of cooked chicken or turkey.

Extras: Add a few tortilla chips, crispy crackers, or pickle sticks. And if you are a "fiercely fastidious finger fooder". . . take a few toothpicks.

To tote: Package dippers and dip separately in prechilled thermos jars or arrange in a compartmented container with a tight seal and add a refrigerant to the lunch kit to keep everything cold.

Hummus Dip

Try this with tortilla chips, pita bread triangles, or raw vegetables.

> 2 cups chick peas, drained (cooked or canned)
> ⅓ cup olive oil
> ⅓ cup fresh lemon juice
> 2 cloves garlic, minced
> 1–2 drops hot pepper sauce
> ¼ cup tahini (sesame paste)

Combine all ingredients, *except tahini,* in jar of blender and blend until smooth. Add tahini; blend again. (If mixture is too thick, add a little of the liquid drained from the chick peas.) Refrigerate several hours or overnight to blend flavors.

To tote, package in prechilled wide mouth thermos jar; package "dippers" separately.

Vegetable Dip

Package this in a small thermos jar and carry a separate bag of crisp, raw vegetables.

1 8-ounce package cream cheese*
½ cup peeled, chopped cucumber
¼ cup peeled and chopped daikon or white radish
1 tablespoon lemon juice
½ tablespoon prepared mustard

Blend ingredients in blender until smooth, adding 1–3 tablespoons water or apple juice if a thinner consistency is desired.

* Drained and crumbled tofu may be substituted for part of the cream cheese.

Ham Dip

This is particularly nice with crisp celery or carrot sticks and wedges of sweet green pepper.

³/₄ cup diced ham
½ small onion
½ cup mayonnaise
1 tablespoon Worcestershire sauce
⅛ teaspoon ground cloves
⅛ teaspoon nutmeg

Place all ingredients in jar of electric blender; cover and blend until smooth.

To vary, substitute part or all of the mayonnaise with cottage cheese or tofu. Adjust seasonings to taste.

Chili Bean Dip

This low fat dip contains only 17 calories per tablespoon.

1 16-ounce can red kidney beans, drained
1 tablespoon vinegar
¾ teaspoon chili powder
¼ teaspoon salt
1 tablespoon minced onion
1 teaspoon dried parsley

Place drained beans in blender jar with vinegar, chili powder, and salt. Blend until smooth. Stir in onion and parsley. Chill well.

Tangy Seafood Dunk

1 cup egg or *tofu mayonnaise*
1/4 cup catsup
1 tablespoon chili sauce
2 teaspoons horseradish
1 tablespoon lemon juice
1 clove garlic, minced
1/8 teaspoon Tabasco sauce

Mix all ingredients until smooth. Chill for several hours to blend flavors.

Vary the flavor by substituting 2 teaspoons minced pickle or bottled capers for the horseradish.

Orange Blossom Dip for Fruit

Delectable with strawberries, chunks of pineapple or other seasonal fruit.

1 8-ounce package light cream cheese or 1 cup yogurt cheese,
    page 52
1/4 cup fresh orange juice
1 teaspoon grated orange peel
2 tablespoons sugar

Combine ingredients in jar of electric blender; cover and whiz until smooth. Chill.

Spicy Cream Dip

Try this one scooped up with slices of chilled pears.

1 cup sour cream or yogurt cheese, page 52
2 tablespoons milk (if using yogurt cheese)
2 tablespoons brown sugar
1/2 teaspoon cinnamon

In small bowl, combine all ingredients; mix well. Chill.

Creamy Molded Chicken Salad

Beautifully cooling on a warm day.

> 1 8¼-ounce can crushed pineapple
> ½ cup chicken broth
> 1 tablespoon (1 envelope) unflavored gelatin
> ⅓ cup pineapple juice (drained from pineapple)
> ½ cup mayonnaise
> ⅓ cup plain yogurt
> 1 cup diced cooked chicken
> 1 teaspoon grated onion
> ½ teaspoon salt
> ¼ cup diced celery
> ½ cup diced oranges or seedless grapes
> ¼ cup slivered almonds

Drain pineapple, *reserving liquid*. Combine gelatin and chicken broth in small saucepan; let stand one minute. Stir over medium heat until gelatin is dissolved; add pineapple juice. Cool. Stir together mayonnaise and yogurt; gradually add cooled gelatin mixture. Fold in remaining ingredients. Turn into a 6-cup mold or shallow square dish and refrigerate until firm. Nice served on a bed of romaine or shredded lettuce.

To tote, carry in prechilled thermos jar; tote shredded lettuce separately, if desired.

Fancy Fruit Salad

Good plain or with yogurt, tofu, or cottage cheese.

> 2 cups each: strawberries, stems removed
>   fresh or canned pineapple chunks
>   cantaloupe cubes or orange sections
>   seedless grapes
> Juice and grated rind from: 1 orange
>   1 lemon
>   1 lime
> ½ cup maple syrup or corn syrup

Bring ingredients other than fruits to a boil. Pour over prepared fruit. Marinate in a covered container, refrigerated, one hour. Keeps 3 days.

To tote, package in prechilled wide mouth thermos jar.

Springtime Vegetable Mold

2 tablespoons (2 envelopes) unflavored gelatin
2 tablespoons honey or sugar (optional)
1 ½ cups boiling water
1 cup mayonnaise
¼ cup favorite Italian or Cream Cheese Herb Dressing
3 tablespoons lemon juice
2 cups chopped or diced raw vegetables: asparagus, broccoli,
*   celery, mushrooms, tomatoes, and/or zucchini*

In large bowl, mix gelatin with sugar (if using); add boiling water and stir until gelatin is completely dissolved. With whisk, blend in mayonnaise, dressing and lemon juice. Chill, stirring occasionally, until mixture is consistency of unbeaten egg whites. Fold in desired vegetables. Turn into an 8-inch round or square pan; chill until firm. Cut into squares and serve.

To tote: carry in prechilled thermos jar.

Carrot and Pineapple Salad

A standard favorite that is especially popular with children.

1 tablespoon (1 envelope) unflavored gelatin
2 tablespoons honey or sugar
1 ½ cups apple juice, cider, or orange juice
1 ½ cups grated carrots
1 8-ounce can crushed pineapple
1 tablespoon lemon juice
Pinch of salt

In medium bowl, mix gelatin with sugar (if using). Heat ½ cup of the juice to boiling; add to gelatin and stir until gelatin is completely dissolved. Stir in remaining ingredients. Pour into 1-quart mold or shallow square dish and chill until firm.

To tote, pack in prechilled thermos jar.

Cranberry Apple Waldorf

2 tablespoons (2 envelopes) unflavored gelatin
2 tablespoons honey or sugar
1 cup boiling water or apple juice
2 cups cranberry juice cocktail
1 cup chopped apple
¼ cup chopped celery
½ cup chopped nuts

In medium bowl, mix gelatin with sugar (if using). Add boiling water and stir until gelatin is completely dissolved. Stir in cranberry juice. Chill, stirring occasionally, until mixture is consistency of unbeaten egg whites. Fold in remaining ingredients. Turn into mold or shallow square dish and chill until firm.

To tote, pack in prechilled thermos jar.

Spicy Applesauce Mold

½ cup apple juice
1 tablespoon (1 envelope) unflavored gelatin
3 tablespoons red cinnamon candy
2 cups applesauce
¼ teaspoon nutmeg
1 teaspoon lemon juice

Sprinkle gelatin over apple juice in small saucepan; let stand a few minutes. Heat, stirring, until gelatin is completely dissolved. Remove from heat and stir in candies, stirring until dissolved. Stir in remaining ingredients. Turn into small mold and chill until firm.

To tote, pack in prechilled thermos jar.

Enhance the flavor of lunch box salads with the fresh flavor of home-made salad dressing. Package in 2-ounce mini plastic containers or save small spice jars or flavoring bottles for that use.

Basic Salad Dressing and Variations

½ teaspoon salt
⅛ teaspoon pepper
1 tablespoon sugar or honey
¼ cup salad vinegar
¾ cup oil

Combine dry ingredients in jar; mix well. Add remaining ingredients; shake well. Chill.

Creamy French: Add 1 teaspoon dry mustard, ½ teaspoon basil, 1 clove garlic, 1 teaspoon tomato paste, and 2 tablespoons mayonnaise. Blend in electric blender until smooth.

Punchy Blue: Add ¼ cup crumbled Roquefort or blue cheese to Basic Dressing. Blend in electric blender until smooth.

Ruby Red: Add 1 teaspoon *each* thyme, marjoram, and dill weed; 1 bay leaf, pinch *each* tarragon and paprika, 2 tablespoons tomato paste. Shake well.

Zesty Italian: Add 1 teaspoon oregano, 1 small bay leaf, and 1 clove crushed garlic. Shake well.

Almond Dressing

½ cup chopped almonds
2 cloves garlic
¾ cup oil
¼ cup wine vinegar
½ teaspoon salt

Place all ingredients in jar of electric blender; cover, and whiz until smooth and creamy. Refrigerate. Particularly good on tossed green salad.

Creamy Green Dressing

1 cup egg or tofu mayonnaise
½ cup minced greens (watercress, spinach, chives, etc.)
1–2 cloves garlic
¼ teaspoon salt
⅛ teaspoon dry mustard

Place all ingredients in jar of electric blender; cover, and whiz until smooth and creamy. Refrigerate.

Sweet and Sour Salad Dressing

⅓ cup vegetable oil
3 tablespoons apple cider vinegar
1 teaspoon prepared mustard
1 teaspoon lemon juice
2 teaspoons maple syrup
seeds from 1 pomegranate

Combine ingredients in small jar and shake until well blended. Good over plain tossed salad or cooked grains.

Low Calorie Italian Dressing

Only 16 calories per tablespoon.

1 tablespoon rice*
¾ cup water
¼ teaspoon salt
¼ cup mild vinegar
1 small clove garlic, minced
1 teaspoon sugar
2 tablespoons oil
Salt and pepper to taste
1 small bayleaf

Bring water and salt to boil; add rice. Reduce heat; boil, covered, 45 minutes or until rice is mushy. Measure; add cold water until rice and water mixture measures ¾ cup. Pour into blender jar; add vinegar, garlic, oregano, and sugar. Cover and blend at highest speed until mixture is completely smooth. Remove blender jar top and with blender at medium-low speed, gradually add oil until blended in. Add salt and pepper, if desired. Pour into jar containing bay leaf. Chill well. Shake well before using.

* Use glutinous rice (available from oriental groceries), if possible. Or, 2 tablespoons instant rice may be substituted if desired; reduce boiling time to 15 minutes or until rice is mushy.

Fresh Strawberry Dressing

The perfect dressing for fruit salads or fruit-dipping.

¾ cup sliced ripe strawberries
2 tablespoons light corn syrup or honey
½ cup mayonnaise or tofu mayonnaise

Mash strawberries together with corn syrup or honey. Add mayonnaise or tofu mayonnaise, stirring until well blended. Chill.

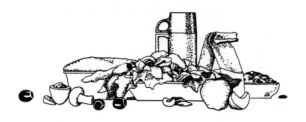

7: Great Go-withs and Saucy Seasonings

Crackers and Crunchies
Side Dishes
Savory Stuff

Gone are the days when spicy sauces existed only to mask the flavor of rotting meats or rancid oils. While the availability of fresher ingredients has done away with the "need," we still appreciate a tangy accompaniment to tickle the palate. Who doesn't enjoy a few crunchy nibbles . . . a savory sauce. . . a flavor "surprise" to round out a meal? A crisp pickle or a handful of potato chips. . . a splash of barbecue sauce or a dollop of hot mustard? But these are among the hardest commercial foods to select from the supermarket shelf. While some are processed only with fine, fresh ingredients, others contain artificial coloring, sugar, excess salt, stabilizers, and preservatives. Only a close inspection of the label will tell. (Maybe! Some chemical additives used in standard recipes do not have to appear on the label.)

What the label will tell you unmistakably us the price. And it's no secret that the "small" mealtime luxuries are often the "big" ticket items in the shopping cart. An ounce of potato chips for the price of a pound of fresh potatoes, a twelve ounce box of crackers for the price of a five pound bag of flour, or an eight ounce jar of pickles for the price of a quart of fresh, sliced pickles; these are high premiums you can avoid if you have the time to make your own. (Even if you don't *have* the time, you may find it worth *making* the little time it takes.)

Honied Graham Crackers

Great plain or with peanut butter, honey, or cream cheese and pine-apple sandwich filling for a nutritious snack.

½ cup margarine, softened
¼ cup honey
1 cup maple syrup
3 cups whole-wheat flour (or use half unbleached all-purpose
    flour)
1 teaspoon baking powder
½ teaspoon baking soda

Cream margarine until light; beat in honey and maple syrup until blended. Mix in dry ingredients. Chill until firm enough to roll out (about ½–1 hour in freezer).

Preheat oven 350°. Divide batter in half. Roll* each half into a 10″ × 15″ rectangle. Cut each rectangle onto 10 5 × 2½-inch crackers. Make perforated lines through the centers with a fork. Place on lightly greased cookie sheets. Bake 8–10 minutes. Remove to wire racks to cool. Makes 20.

*Maple syrup makes a soft dough. An easy way to roll these out is to roll out on waxed paper and then transfer the waxed paper and dough to the cookie sheet. After baking, peel off the waxed paper.

Nutty Rye Crackers

⅓ cup oil, preferably corn oil
⅔ cup water
¼ teaspoon salt
1 cup rolled rye or oatmeal
1 cup whole-wheat flour
½ cup rye flour
⅔ cup crushed coarsely ground walnuts, preferably roasted first

Preheat oven to 375°. Combine oil, water, and salt in a medium-size bowl until blended. Stir in remaining ingredients until mixture forms a ball. Roll out between two sheets of waxed paper or on a lightly floured board until ⅛–¼″ thick. Cut with cookie cutters or into squares or diamonds. Place on cookie sheets which have been sprinkled with cornmeal. Bake 10–20 minutes (depending on size and thickness). Let cool on wire racks.

Vegetable Wheat Thins

Crisp, flavorful little crackers that go together in a jiffy.

> ¼ cup dried vegetable flakes
> 1 tablespoon minced onion
> ½ teaspoon each: celery salt
>   dried parsley flakes
>   oregano
>   thyme or savory
> ½ cup plain yogurt
> 1 tablespoon honey
> 1 cup unbleached all-purpose flour
> ¾ cup whole-wheat flour
> ¼ teaspoon baking soda
> ¼ teaspoon salt
> ⅓ cup real mayonnaise

Preheat oven to 400°. In electric blender (or with mortar and pestle), grind vegetable flakes and onion until pulverized. Add herbs and grind a bit more to release flavors of herbs. Stir into yogurt and honey and let stand while preparing remaining ingredients. In medium bowl, thoroughly stir together flours, baking soda, and salt. With a pastry blender, cut in mayonnaise until well mixed and coarse crumbs form. With fork, stir in yogurt mixture. Press dough firmly into a ball; cut into 3 pieces and shape each into a flattened ball.

Place each ball of dough on an ungreased large cookie sheet. Cover with a sheet of waxed paper and roll to approximately 10 × 15 inches (dough should be *very* thin). Carefully peel off waxed paper. Trim ragged edges but leave trimmings in place. Cut in 1½-inch squares; cut again in triangles, if desired. Prick with fork all over; sprinkle lightly with additional salt. Bake on middle oven shelf 6–8 minutes or until lightly browned. Remove to wire racks to cool completely before storing in tightly covered container.

Easy Bread Sticks

Tuck a few of these into the lunch box with a Chef's Salad.

> 1 1-pound loaf whole-wheat bread
> ⅓ cup oil, preferably corn or sunflower
> ⅓ cup margarine (or additional oil)
> 1 teaspoon Italian seasoning
> 1 teaspoon rosemary
> ¼ teaspoon dry mustard
> ¼ teaspoon paprika
> ¼ teaspoon salt

Preheat oven to 400°. Remove crusts from bread, if desired. Making stacks of 5 or 6 slices, cut into "sticks" about ½-inch wide. Melt margarine, if using, and combine with all remaining ingredients. Place bread "sticks" on greased cookie sheets. Drizzle oil mixture over. Bake 15–20 minutes, turning once halfway through. Let cool on wire racks. Store in covered container if not eating immediately.

Crunchy Croutons

Every good green salad deserves a topping of these flavorful bits.

> 4 cups ¼-inch cubes fresh bread (about 5 slices white and
>   3 slices rye or whole-wheat)
> 2 tablespoons salad oil
> 1 tablespoon dried parsley
> ¾ teaspoon garlic salt
> ½ teaspoon each: oregano
>   paprika
> ¼ teaspoon each: thyme
>   basil
>   pepper

Preheat oven to 300°. Toast bread crumbs in shallow baking pan or cookie sheet for 30 minutes. Cool slightly. Drizzle with oil; stir in spices, mixing well. Cool completely before storing in airtight containers.

Busy Day Tip: Crunchy Croutons make a good substitute for packaged bread stuffing.

Savory Add-a-Crunch

From the creative cooks at The Quaker Oats Company, here is a nutritious substitute for croutons. This adds a flavorful crunch wherever you use it—over tossed green salads, soups, casseroles or vegetables.

> 2 cups Quaker Oats (Quick or Old Fashioned, uncooked)
> ½ cup butter or margarine, melted
> ⅓ cup grated Parmesan cheese
> ⅓ cup wheat germ, unprocessed bran or chopped nuts
>   (optional)
> ¼ teaspoon onion or garlic salt
> 1 teaspoon oregano leaves and ½ teaspoon thyme leaves
>   (optional)

Preheat oven to 350°. Combine all ingredients; mix well. Bake in ungreased 15½ × 10½-inch jelly roll pan 15–18 minutes or until light golden brown. Cool; store in tightly covered container in refrigerator up to 3 months. Makes about 3 cups.

Tortilla Chips

Good hot or cold, these are great to carry as "scoops" for foods like ratatouille or chili—much more fun than using a spoon!

6 corn tortillas
¼ teaspoon salt

Preheat oven to 400°. Cut each tortilla into 5 or 6 pie-shaped wedges. Place wedges on ungreased cookie sheet and sprinkle evenly with salt. Bake 10 minutes; turn over with spatula and bake 2–3 minutes longer. Cool slightly on wire racks or paper towels. Good plain or with dip.

Potato Skin Munchies

Leftover baked potato skins
Oil
Salt (optional)
Paprika, oregano, or rosemary

Preheat oven to 450°. Cut skins into 1-inch wide strips. Brush lightly with oil and spinkle with seasoning, if desired. Bake until crisp, about 7–8 minutes.

Nutty Nibbles

1 cup peanuts
1 cup walnuts
1 cup sunflower seeds
1 cup almonds
1 tablespoon tamari or soy sauce
1 tablespoon oil

Preheat oven to 300°. Combine all ingredients and spread on two greased cookie sheets. Bake 15 minutes. Cool completely before storing in covered container or plastic bags.

Spicy Seeds

Great for just snacking or as a spicy "extra" in a brown bag.

1 cup pumpkin seeds
2 tablespoons oil
1 tablespoon tamari orsoy sauce
¼ teaspoon chili powder
½ clove garlic, crushed and minced

Preheat oven to 300°. Combine ingredients and spread on a cookie sheet. Bake about 10 minutes or until seeds are golden brown. Cool before storing in tightly covered container or plastic bags.

Roasted Soy Nuts

Rinse and pick over soybeans, discarding any damaged or broken beans. Soak *each* cup of dry soybeans in 4 cups of water overnight in a cool spot.

Preheat oven to 200°. Drain soybeans well, dry, and place in single layer on cookie sheet(s). Bake 2 hours. Salt while warm, if desired. Cool completely before storing in covered containers.

Nuts: Toasted and Roasted

Plain Toasted Nuts:

1-4 cups whole or chopped nuts

Preheat oven to 350°. Spread nuts evenly on cookie sheet(s). Bake 10 minutes, stirring the nuts after 5 minutes. Remove from oven and allow to cool before packaging in airtight containers.

Plain Roasted Nuts:

Follow the directions for Plain Toasted Nuts *except* grease each cookie sheet with 1 tablespoon oil before baking.

Tamari Roasted Nuts:

2 cups whole or chopped nuts
1 tablespoon tamari or soy sauce
1 tablespoon oil

Combine the nuts and tamari or soy sauce in a small bowl. Grease cookie sheet with oil and bake as for Plain Toasted Nuts.

Crunchy Roasted Nuts:

2 cups chopped nuts
2 tablespoons sesame seeds
2 tablespoons sesame oil

Combine ingredients, spread on cookie sheet and bake as for Plain Toasted Nuts.

Sweet Roasted Nuts:

1 cup whole almonds
2 tablespoons soft margarine or oil
½ cup maple syrup

Combine ingredients, spread on cookie sheet and bake as for Plain Toasted Nuts. (These may take a few minutes longer but check them occasionally because they burn more easily than the others.) Let cool and break apart if stuck together.

Ruby Applesauce

A nice compliment to a peanut butter or ham sandwich on whole-wheat bread. Great for pancakes or plain cake.

8 cups peeled, sliced apples
1 ½ cups cranberries, left whole or halved
¾ – 1 cup maple syrup
2 tablespoons lemon juice
½ cup apple juice or water

Combine all ingredients in a large saucepan. Bring to a boil, lower heat, cover, and simmer until tender, about 10–15 minutes. Serve warm or chilled. (Applesauce will thicken as it cools.)

Pickled Beets

Save the leftover juice for Pickled Pink Eggs.

2 1-pound jars sliced beets
1 small onion, thinly sliced
½ cup apple cider vinegar
½ cup maple syrup
¼ teaspoon cloves
¼ teaspoon allspice
½ cup reserved beet liquid

Drain beets, reserving ½ cup of the liquid. Combine beets and onions in large bowl. Combine all remaining ingredients in saucepan; bring to boil. Pour over beets and onions; cover and chill.

Carrot Pickle Sticks

Carrots (enough to fill quart jar)
1 cup white wine vinegar or apple cider vinegar
1 cup maple syrup
1 cup water
½ cup apple juice
1 tablespoon mustard seed
½ red pepper, slivered
2–3 sprigs fresh dill

Wash, pare and cut sufficient carrots into sticks to fill a quart jar (a sterilized, used pickle jar works well). Bring remaining ingredients to a boil and pour over carrots. Cap; refrigerate at least 3 days before using.

Ever-ready Coleslaw

Don't shudder at all the sugar in this recipe! Most of the calories are discarded when you drain the marinade from the salad before serving.

1 2-pound head cabbage, shredded
1 medium onion, chopped
1 medium green pepper, chopped
1 tablespoon salt
1 cup vinegar
1½ cups sugar*
1 teaspoon celery seed
½ teaspoon mustard seed

Combine vegetables and salt in large pan. Pour boiling water over to cover; cover and let stand for one hour. Drain well and return to pan. Heat vinegar, sugar, and spices in small saucepan until sugar dissolves. Pour over vegetables; mix well. Store in glass container in refrigerator. Let flavors blend for a day before serving. Keeps for several weeks in refrigerator.

*Substituting maple syrup will make a "soupy"—but still tasty—salad.

Deluxe Devilled Eggs

6 eggs, hardcooked and peeled
1 tablespoon each: mayonnaise
                    soft margarine
                    plain yogurt
1 teaspoon each: Parmesan cheese
                  Worcestershire sauce
                  onion juice

Cut eggs in half lengthwise and remove yolks. Mash the yolks well; then stir in remaining ingredients until smooth. Spoon back into egg white halves. Garnish with a sprinkling of paprika, if desired. Refrigerate, covered.

Tote neatly by reassembling the halves and wrapping in plastic wrap.

Duxelle Devilled Eggs

6 eggs, hardcooked and shelled
¼ cup Duxelles, page 125
1 tablespoon each: mayonnaise
                    soft margarine
                    minced chives
                    white wine or tamari sauce

Cut eggs in half lengthwise and remove yolks. Mash the yolks well; then stir in remaining ingredients. Spoon back into egg white halves. Store or package as above.

Pickled Pink Eggs

These are pretty sliced and served on a bed of greens.

6 eggs, hardcooked and shelled
leftover pickling liquid from pickled beets, page 123

Pour liquid over the eggs in a jar or bowl. Cover and marinate in refrigerator 1–3 days. Drain to serve or package for toting.

Duxelles

Freeze small containers of Duxelles for adding to omelet fillings, stuffings, salads or sauces.

2 tablespoons butter or margarine
8-10 ounces fresh mushrooms, minced
¼ cup finely minced onion
1 tablespoon minced parsley
½ teaspoon salt

Heat butter or margarine in heavy frying pan. Add remaining ingredients; sauté over medium heat 5–7 minutes, stirring constantly, until moisture has evaporated. (Add more butter if needed.) Store, covered in refrigerator up to 7–10 days or freeze.

Sweet Pickles Today

Almost "instant" pickles, these are ready as soon as they are chilled.

½ cup cider vinegar
¼ cup water
¼ cup honey or granulated sugar
½ teaspoon salt
½ teaspoon mustard seed
¼ teaspoon celery seed
Dash turmeric
1 medium or 2 small cucumbers, sliced (about 2½ cups)
1 small onion, thinly sliced

Combine all ingredients, *except* cucumber and onion, in medium-size saucepan. Stirring constantly, heat to boiling and cook for 5 minutes. Add cucumber and onion; simmer 10 minutes or until cucumbers are tender but still crisp. Cover; let stand 10 minutes. Pour into container, cover, and chill before serving. Keeps several days in refrigerator.

Half Dills Tomorrow

Make these for lunch the next day.

½ *cup cider vinegar*
½ *cup water*
2 *tablespoons sugar or* honey
¼ *teaspoon salt*
½ *teaspoon dillweed*
1 *large or 2 medium cucumbers, thinly sliced (about 3 cups)*
1 *small clove garlic, minced*

Prepare as for *Sweet Pickles Today* above.

Budget Minded Sweet Pickles

Beat the higher cost of sweet pickles by using this little trick for making your own.

1 *1-quart jar whole dill pickles* (not *Kosher or garlic-flavored*)
½ - ¾ *cup sugar (or preferred sweetener)*
1 *teaspoon celery seed*

Drain pickles and slice into thin rounds. Into a wide-mouthed jar that has a leak-proof screw cap, layer the pickles, sprinkling each layer with some of the sugar and celery seed. Cap tightly and let stand for a day, turning the jar occasionally, before refrigerating. For best flavor, wait a few days before eating.

Onion-Pepper Relish

Good warm or cold.

4 *onions, chopped*
1 *green pepper, chopped*
1 *red pepper, chopped*
½ *cup cranberry-apple juice*
¼ *cup honey*
¼ *cup apple cider vinegar*
1 *tablespoon prepared mustard*
2 *teaspoons horseradish*
2 *teaspoons salt*
2 *tablespoons oil or margarine*

Combine all ingredients in a saucepan. Bring to boil. Lower heat; cook ½ hour, stirring several times. Store in a large jar or covered container in refrigerator. Stays fresh for at least 10 days. Makes about 2½ cups.

Catsup

If you use a lot of catsup, this recipe provides a good way to reduce sugar and preservatives in your diet.

1 28-ounce can tomatoes in puree
1 6-ounce can tomato paste
2 large onions, chopped
2–3 tablespoons honey or brown sugar
2 tablespoons vinegar, preferably apple cider
¼ teaspoon each: dry mustard
                paprika
                Tabasco sauce

Place all ingredients in jar of blender; cover and whiz until smooth. (You may have to do this in two batches.) Pour into a heavy saucepan. Bring to a boil; lower heat and simmer, uncovered, about 2 hours, stirring occasionally. Pour into glass jars and refrigerate while still hot. Will stay fresh for at least one month.

Chili Sauce

1 28-ounce can tomatoes in puree, undrained but chopped
1½ cups chopped onion
1 cup chopped red and/or green pepper
⅓ cup honey or maple syrup
½ cup apple cider vinegar
½ teaspoon salt
¼ teaspoon each: black pepper
                ground cloves
                allspice
⅛ teaspoon cayenne pepper

Mix all ingredients in heavy saucepan. Cook over low heat, uncovered, 1½–2 hours, stirring occasionally. Store in covered glass jars in refrigerator.

No-Salt Seasoning

Try this in your salt shaker. Even the kids are not too young to learn to cut down on salt.

¼ cup sesame seeds
½ teaspoon dry mustard
½ teaspoon paprika
1 teaspoon each: oregano, basil, and thyme

Mix all ingredients in a blender or mortar and pestle and grind until pulverized. Use as a table or cooking seasoning.

Sweet and Sour Sauce

This is good served over warm or cold slices of leftover bean, grain, or chicken loaf.

2 tablespoons oil or margarine
¼ cup maple syrup
2 tablespoons water
2 tablespoons apple cider vinegar
1 vegetable or chicken broth cube
¼ teaspoon salt
½ teaspoon tamari or Worcestershire sauce

Combine all ingredients in small saucepan; bring to boil and simmer 7–8 minutes. Pour or brush over warm or cold loaf slices; sprinkle with minced scallions, if desired.

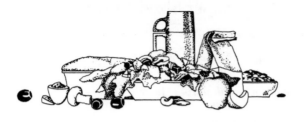

8: Naturally Good Totable Treats

Cookies
Pastries
Cakes
Confections

We have developed such "sophisticated" tastes we have lost our ancestors' appreciation of the bounty of "treats" nature has provided. Mother Earth offered, and early man indulged in, cherries and apples. He enjoyed them fresh, in season, and dried as winter treats. Later Mediterraneans enjoyed a variety of fruits: apples, apricots, dates, figs, melons, pears, and plums. Ancients in the Mid-Eastern lands feasted on cakes and yogurts with a variety of fresh and dried fruits. The Persians mixed fruits with nuts, honey, and spices or baked thin, flaky pastry with honey and nuts. For dessert, Romans stuffed dates with nuts and pine kernels and fried them with honey. Or they indulged in African sweet-wine cakes with honey.

Honey was the basic sweetener throughout early history. Sugar was introduced to Europe in the eighth century when the Moors planted cane in Spain, but it remained a rare luxury until sugar cane was grown cheaply in the New World. By the end of the eighteenth century, a process for producing sugar from beets had been developed that further increased the affordability of sugar for the common man.

Historically, then, our romance with refined sugar has indeed been a short one. Statements by nutritionists opposed to the use of too much sugar are encouraging us to rediscover the natural pleasures of desserts enhanced by fruits, nuts, and honey—the sweets originally, and naturally, provided by Mother Earth.

[129]

Super Sized Cookies

Easy to make; easy to take.

Basic Dough:

1 cup unbleached all-purpose flour
1 cup whole-wheat flour
¾ cup soft margarine or ⅔ cup oil
½ cup brown sugar
1-2 eggs (1 egg makes a more fragile cookie)
½ teaspoon salt

Cream margarine until fluffy; beat in sweeteners and egg(s) until creamy. Stir in remaining ingredients until smooth. Drop by ⅓ cupfuls, 5 to a lightly greased cookie sheet; flatten to a 3–4-inch circle with wet hands. Bake as directed in variations. Each recipe makes about 1 dozen cookies.

Variations:

Chocolate Chip— Add to basic dough:
        ½ cup additional all-purpose flour
        ½ cup maple syrup
        2 teaspoons vanilla
        1 cup chocolate chips
        1 cup chopped nuts
        Preheat oven to 375°. Bake 14–15 minutes.

Carrot Granola— Add to basic dough:
        ½ cup honey
        1 ⅓ cups grated carrots
        1 ⅓ cups granola
        1 teaspoon baking powder
        ½ teaspoon nutmeg
        1 teaspoon vanilla
        1 teaspoon lemon extract
        Preheat oven to 350°. Bake 13–14 minutes.

Joe Froggers—   Add to basic dough:
        ½ cup molasses
        1 teaspoon ginger
        ½ teaspoon allspice
        ¼ teaspoon nutmeg
        ½ teaspoon baking soda
        ¼ cup rum, brandy, or black coffee
        Preheat oven to 350°. (Drop these by ¼-cupfuls, 5 to a sheet.) Bake 15–16 minutes.

Oat Crunchies— Add to basic dough:
¼ cup margarine
⅔ cup honey or *brown sugar*
2 cups oatmeal
½ teaspoon baking soda
Plus this: 1½ cups raisins
1 tablespoon cinnamon
1 tablespoon grated orange rind
Or this: 1½ cups chopped almonds or coconut
1 teaspoon lemon extract
2 tablespoons grated lemon rind
Preheat oven to 350°. Bake 14–15 minutes.

Peanut Butter— Reduce margarine to ½ cup
Add to basic dough:
½ cup peanut butter
½ cup honey or *brown sugar*
1 teaspoon baking powder
1 teaspoon almond or *vanilla extract*
Preheat oven to 350°. Bake 14–15 minutes.

Busy Day Tip: Freeze pre-shaped ⅓ cupfuls of batter; bake as directed when desired.

Super Cider Cookies

½ cup apple cider
1 cup currants
¼ cup apple juice concentrate, thawed
¼ cup maple syrup
1 cup margarine, softened
2½ cups whole-wheat flour
½ teaspoon baking powder
¼ teaspoon salt

Combine cider, currants, maple syrup, and apple juice concentrate in a small saucepan and bring to boil. Remove from heat and allow to cool completely.

Preheat oven to 375°. Cream margarine until fluffy. Beat in currant mixture. Stir in remaining ingredients. Form mixture into small balls using 1 tablespoon batter for each. Place on greased cookie sheets. Bake 16–20 minutes. Cool on wire racks.

Bulgur Cookies

1 cup uncooked bulgur
⅔ cup oil, preferably corn oil
½ cup maple syrup
½ cup honey
1 teaspoon baking soda
2 teaspoons baking powder
3 cups whole-wheat or unbleached all-purpose flour
1 tablespoon apple pie spice
1 cup raisins

Soak bulgur in 1 cup hot water for 5–10 minutes or until all water is absorbed. Beat oil and sweeteners together until smooth and creamy. Stir in remaining ingredients. Refrigerate 1–3 hours.

Preheat oven to 350°. Drop batter by tablespoons onto lightly greased cookie sheets. Bake 10 minutes. Let stand on pans for 5 minutes before removing to wire racks to cool. Makes 4–5 dozen.

Peanut Butter Apple Cookies

½ cup margarine, softened
1½ cups whole-wheat or unbleached all-purpose flour
2 teaspoons vanilla
¼ cup apple juice concentrate, thawed
½ cup brown sugar
2 eggs
½ teaspoon baking soda

Preheat oven to 375°. Cream margarine until fluffy. Blend in peanut butter, eggs, vanilla, apple juice, and brown sugar; beat until creamy. Stir in dry ingredients until well mixed. Drop by tablespoonfuls onto greased baking sheets, flattening with a greased glass or by hand. Bake 10 minutes or until done. Remove to wire racks to cool.

Pumpkin Cookies

1½ cups whole-wheat flour
½ teaspoon baking soda
1½ teaspoons baking powder
1 teaspoon cinnamon
¼ teaspoon cloves
¼ teaspoon salt
½ cup margarine
⅓ cup maple syrup or liquid brown sugar
¼ cup apple cider
1 cup pureed pumpkin
2 teaspoons vanilla
1 cup chopped almonds or walnuts

Preheat oven to 350°. Cream margarine until fluffy; beat in maple syrup, cider, vanilla, and pumpkin. Add dry ingredients all at once; stir until well blended. Drop by tablespoons on ungreased baking sheets. Bake 12–15 minutes. Remove to wire racks to cool. Makes 3–4 dozen.

Peanut Butter Scotchies

½ cup corn flake crumbs
½ teaspoon baking powder
¼ teaspoon salt
½ cup coarsely chopped nuts
¼ cup butter or margarine
1 cup light brown sugar, packed
⅓ cup peanut butter
2 eggs, lightly beaten
Confectioners sugar (optional)

Preheat oven to 350°. Combine corn flake crumbs, baking powder, salt and nuts. Set aside. Melt butter; remove from heat. Stir in brown sugar and peanut butter until well combined. Add eggs; beat well. Stir in crumb mixture. Spread in greased 9 × 9 × 2-inch pan. Bake 30 minutes. When cool, cut into squares and roll in confectioners' sugar, if desired. Makes about 25.

Pineapple Bars

Good warm or cold, they derive most of their sweetness from the fruit.

1 15-ounce can unsweetened pineapple, undrained
1⅓ cups peeled, chopped apple
¾ cup brown sugar
1½ cups whole-wheat flour
1 teaspoon baking soda
1 egg
½ teaspoon salt
¼ teaspoon ginger

Preheat oven to 350°. Stir together dry ingredients in a large bowl and set aside. Combine remaining ingredients in a medium bowl, stirring to blend and incorporate egg. Pour over dry ingredients and mix with a fork or wooden spoon until just moistened. Spoon into greased 9 × 13 × 2-inch baking pan. Bake 40 minutes. Cool in pan on wire rack before cutting into squares.

Add punch when serving this at home by serving warm with a dollop of sour cream—slightly sweetened with brown sugar.

Spicy Apple Bars

1 cup whole-wheat flour
½ cup Nutri-grain Corn cereal (crushed to ¼ cup)
1 teaspoon baking soda
½ teaspoon cinnamon
1 cup firmly packed brown sugar
2 cups chopped, peeled apples
½ cup chopped nuts
⅓ cup oil

Preheat oven to 350°. Combine flour, cereal, baking soda, cinnamon, and salt in a large bowl. Stir in sugar, apples, and nuts. Beat egg and oil together until well blended; stir into flour-apple mixture until mixture is evenly moistened. (Batter will be stiff.) Turn into greased 8-inch square baking pan. Bake 35 minutes or until center springs back when lightly pressed. Cool in pan on wire rack before cutting into bars. Makes 12.

Fruit Bars

Substitute dried apricots, pears or other dried fruit for the raisins.

1 cup currants or seedless raisins, chopped
½ cup apple or orange juice
1 tablespoon fresh lemon juice
2 tablespoons granulated sugar or maple syrup
¼ cup finely chopped walnuts
½ cup softened margarine
½ cup firmly packed brown sugar
1 teaspoon vanilla
1 teaspoon baking powder
1 cup regular oatmeal
¾ cup whole-wheat flour
½ cup finely chopped walnuts

Preheat oven to 350°. Combine raisins, juices, and granulated sugar in small saucepan; cook over medium heat, stirring until thickened, about 6–7 minutes. Stir in the ¼ cup nuts. Set aside. Cream margarine, brown sugar, and vanilla until light and fluffy. Beat in baking powder. Stir in remaining ingredients. Pat half the mixture into bottom of a greased 8-inch square baking pan. Spread with reserved raisin mixture. Sprinkle with remaining oatmeal mixture. Bake 25–30 minutes. Cool in pan on wire rack. Cut into bars.

Carob Chip Bars

1 cup soft margarine
1 cup maple syrup or *brown sugar*
1 cup carob chips
1 cup chopped walnuts
1 cup whole-wheat flour
1 cup unbleached all-purpose flour
1 teaspoon vanilla

Preheat oven to 350°. Cream margarine until fluffy; beat in syrup or sugar until creamy. Stir in remaining ingredients. Spread in greased jellyroll (10 × 15 × 1-inch) pan. Bake 30 minutes. Cool in pan 5 minutes; cut into squares; continue cooling before removing from pan.

One Bowl Brownies

⅓ cup carob powder or *cocoa*
½ cup unbleached all-purpose flour
¼ teaspoon baking powder
½ cup oil
1 cup brown sugar
2 eggs
1½ teaspoons vanilla
1 cup chopped nuts (optional)

Preheat oven to 350°. Dump everything into a mixing bowl and stir with wooden spoon until well combined. Turn into a greased 9-inch square baking pan. Bake 20–23 minutes or until barely dry to the touch. Cool in pan; cut into bars.

Apple Nut Bars

½ cup margarine
½ cup brown sugar
¼ cup honey
1 egg
1 cup flour, preferably whole-wheat
½ cup baking soda
¼ teaspoon cinnamon
¼ teaspoon ginger
2 apples, peeled, cored, and chopped
¾ cup chopped nuts

Beat margarine, brown sugar, honey, and egg until creamy. Stir in dry ingredients; fold in apples and nuts. Spoon into greased 8-inch square pan. Bake 45 minutes. Cool and store, covered, in pan.

Peanut Butter Granola Bars

2 cups Apple Granola, page 30
⅓ cup peanut butter
¼ cup honey
½ teaspoon vanilla
1 egg

Preheat oven to 350°. Mix all ingredients together well. Spoon into a well-greased 8- or 9-inch square pan, smoothing with damp hands. Bake ½ hour. Cool 15 minutes; cut into bars. Finish cooling before removing from pan. Wrap individual bars in plastic wrap to store.

Fantastic Fig Bars

These really are fantastic and they keep well, covered or frozen.

1 cup margarine, softened
½ cup each: honey and brown sugar
2 egg yolks
1½ teaspoons baking powder
4 cups flour, preferably whole-wheat
2 cups fresh or moist-dried figs, snipped into small pieces
1¼ cups apple juice or water
½ cup honey
Juice and grated rind of 1 lemon
2 tablespoons cornstarch

Cream margarine until fluffy. Beat in sweeteners and egg yolks. Stir in baking powder and flour until well mixed. Form into a ball; wrap in plastic wrap. Chill in freezer 1–4 hours.

Meanwhile, prepare filling. Combine all remaining ingredients, *except* cornstarch, in small saucepan and cook 15 minutes, stirring often. Mix cornstarch with a bit of water, then stir into fig mixture. Cook and stir until clear, less than 1 minute. Cool to room temperature before using.

Preheat oven to 400°. Roll chilled dough into five 6″ × 16″ strips. Spread filling evenly over strips leaving ¼″ margin on one long side and 2½″ on the other long side. Bring edges together and crimp. With a fork, make lines 1½″ apart down the strips. Place on greased cookie sheets and bake 10 minutes. Cool on racks. Cut apart on perforated lines.

Jelly Bars

A satisfying sandwich cookie that you can cut to just the right size for individual appetites.

½ cup margarine
½ cup brown sugar
1 egg yolk
½ cup ground almonds or walnuts
½ teaspoon cinnamon
¾ cup flour, preferably whole-wheat
1 egg white, beaten to soft peaks
¼ cup chopped almonds or walnuts
½ cup jelly (strawberry or currant is good)

Preheat oven to 350°. Beat margarine, brown sugar, and egg with electric mixer until creamy. Stir in next three ingredients. Divide in half. Pat each half into a greased 8-inch square baking pan. Spread beaten egg white and nuts over one pan; leave the other plain. Bake 20 minutes. Cool a few minutes before turning out of pans. Spread jelly on the plain layer; top with the other layer (nuts side up) and cut into squares.

Banana Energy Bars

¾ cup soft butter or margarine
1 cup dark brown sugar, packed
1 egg
½ teaspoon salt
1½ cups mashed ripe bananas
4 cups uncooked regular oatmeal
1 cup raisins
½ cup chopped walnuts

Preheat oven to 350°. Cream butter and sugar until light and fluffy. Beat in egg, salt, and bananas. Stir in remaining ingredients. Turn into greased 13 × 9 × 2-inch baking pan. Bake 1 hour or until cake tester comes out clean. Cool completely before cutting into 2 × 1-inch bars.

Honey Almond Granola Bars

½ cup margarine
¼ cup corn oil
¾ cup honey
½ cup brown sugar
2 cups chopped almonds
3½ cups oatmeal
1 teaspoon vanilla extract
½ teaspoon almond extract

Preheat oven to 450°. In large saucepan, heat margarine, oil, honey and brown sugar until melted. Remove from heat and mix in remaining ingredients. Line a 10 × 15 × 1-inch jellyroll pan with foil or waxed paper. Grease paper well. Spoon in mixture, patting level with wet hands. Bake 10 minutes. Turn out onto rack; peel off paper and let cool completely before cutting into 1½ × 5-inch bars. Makes 20.

Two-layer Brownie Bars

½ cup all-purpose flour
⅛ teaspoon salt
¼ teaspoon baking soda
⅓ cup honey or brown sugar
⅓ cup chopped walnuts
⅓ cup melted margarine or oil
1 cup oatmeal
¾ cup flour
⅛ teaspoon salt
¼ teaspoon baking soda
1 ounce unsweetened chocolate melted with ½ cup margarine
⅔ cup honey or ¾ cup brown sugar
1 egg
Grated rind of 1 orange (optional)

Preheat oven to 350°. Combine first seven ingredients until crumbly. Pat into well-greased 9-inch square (or 7 × 11 × 2-inch) baking pan. Bake 10 minutes.

Meanwhile, mix together the remaining ingredients. Spread over hot, baked crust; return pan to oven and bake 30 minutes longer. Cool in pan before cutting into bars.

Maple Shortbread

1 cup whole-wheat flour
½ cup rye flour
1 cup rolled rye or *oat cereal*
1 cup maple syrup, divided
½ cup margarine, softened
½ cup chopped sunflower seeds or nuts

Preheat oven to 325°. Mix flours, rolled rye, margarine, and ½ cup maple syrup until evenly blended. Pat into a greased 9-inch square (or 11 × 7 × 2-inch) pan. Make shallow, criss-cross lines 1–2 inches apart. Sprinkle with remaining maple syrup and seeds or nuts. Bake 30 minutes. Cook in pan, then cut or break apart on criss-crossed lines.

Apple Butter Pastries

1 package dry yeast
¼ cup warm water (120°)
1 tablespoon honey or *rice syrup*
⅓ cup margarine, softened
1½ cups whole-wheat flour
1½ cups unbleached all-purpose flour
4 egg yolks
½ cup plain yogurt or ⅓ cup soft tofu
Mixture #1:
    2 cups finely chopped walnuts
    ½ cup honey or ⅔ cup rice syrup
    2 teaspoons cinnamon
Mixture #2:
    1¼ cups apple butter
    ½ teaspoon cinnamon
    ½ teaspoon nutmeg

Preheat oven to 350°. Combine first three ingredients and let stand 10–15 minutes. Add next five ingredients and mix until smooth. Divide batter into three balls. Roll out first ball to a 10″ × 14″ rectangle. Place in a lightly greased 9 × 13 × 2-inch pan, turning up all four sides ½″. Spread with Mixture #1. Roll the second ball into a 9″ × 13″ rectangle. Place over the first filling layer and spread with Mixture #2. Roll out the last ball to a 9″ × 13″ rectangle and place over top. Bake 1 hour. Glaze or frost, if desired.

To Glaze: Brush with 2 tablespoons honey or rice syrup while still hot.

To Frost: Beat 4 egg whites with ¼ cup honey or ⅓ cup rice syrup until stiff peaks form. Spread on top of hot pastry. Sprinkle with ⅓ cup finely chopped walnuts, if desired. Bake an additional 15 minutes.

New World Rugelachs

2 cups whole-wheat flour
⅓ cup oil
½ cup margarine, softened
½ cup plain yogurt or crumbled soft tofu
⅔ cup honey or 1 cup rice syrup
1 cup chopped walnuts
1 teaspoon cinnamon

Mix first four ingredients until smooth and well blended. Refrigerate 8-24 hours.

Preheat oven to 400°. Divide batter into four parts. Roll out each piece into a circle (approximately 9-inches in diameter); then cut each circle into six wedges. Combine remaining ingredients to make filling. Sprinkle evenly over wedges. Roll up, beginning at the large end. Place on lightly greased cookie sheets with pointed end down. Bake 20 minutes. Cool on wire racks. Makes 2 dozen.

Apple Dumplings

1 recipe Cheese or Tofu Pastry (page 61)
4 large apples
6 tablespoons maple syrup
2 tablespoons sesame seeds
2 tablespoons currants or minced dried apricots
1 teaspoon cinnamon
2 tablespoons oil

Preheat oven to 350°. Wash, pare, and core apples. Combine 2 tablespoons of the maple syrup and the remaining ingredients; stuff equally into apple centers. Roll out pastry. Cut 4 6-8-inch squares. Center an apple on each square; pull all 4 points of dough up to top of apple and pinch together. Place apples in greased baking dish. Pour remaining 4 tablespoons maple syrup over. Bake 30-35 minutes or until apples are just tender. (Scatter 2 tablespoons additional sesame seeds over after the first 15 minutes of baking, if desired.) Serve warm or cold.

Apple Turnovers

Use the leftover pastry to make Jim Jams another day.

¹/₂ recipe Cheese or Tofu Pastry (page 61)
¹/₂ cups diced apple
¹/₃ cup brown sugar
3 tablespoons all-purpose flour
¹/₂ tablespoons lemon juice
¹/₄ teaspoon cinnamon
¹/₄ teaspoon nutmeg
¹/₈ teaspoon salt

Preheat oven to 425°. Roll pastry ⅛" thick; cut into 4 squares. Combine remaining ingredients; place one-fourth of the filling on each of the pastry squares. Fold in half diagonally and press edges with tines of fork to seal. Slit pastry with sharp knife. Place on ungreased cookie sheet and bake 20–25 minutes.

Jim Jams

These are nutritious enough to serve for breakfast.

Leftover Cheese or Tofu Pastry (page 61)
Cherry or raspberry jam or preserves

Preheat oven to 425°. Roll pastry ⅛-inch thick; cut into 2½-inch squares. Place a teaspoonful of jam or preserves in the center of each square. Fold corners to the center to enclose filling. Place on ungreased cookie sheets. Bake 15 minutes or until lightly browned. Remove to wire racks to cool before sprinkling with confectioners sugar, if desired.

Honey Flake Macaroons

4 egg whites, at room temperature
¹/₂ cup honey
3 cups Corn or Barley Nutri-Grain Flaked Cereal
1 cup chopped almonds or walnuts
1 cup unsweetened flaked coconut

Preheat oven to 300°. Beat egg whites until foamy; add honey, 1 tablespoon at a time and continue beating until very stiff. Gently fold in remaining ingredients. Drop mixture by tablespoonfuls onto lightly greased cookie sheets. Bake 20 minutes. Remove cookies to wire racks to cool. Store covered to keep cookies from getting soggy. Makes about 3 dozen.

Molasses Pumpkin Snack Cake

1 cup whole-wheat flour
1½ cups unbleached all-purpose flour
2 eggs
⅓ cup oil
1 15-ounce can pumpkin
1 cup brown sugar
⅔ cup molasses
½ teaspoon each: allspice
                    nutmeg
                    cinnamon
1 tablespoon baking soda
½ teaspoon baking powder
½ teaspoon salt

Preheat oven to 350°. Combine all ingredients in a large bowl; beat three minutes at medium speed with electric mixer. Turn into greased 9-inch square pan. Bake 45–50 minutes. Cool in pan before cutting into squares.

Add punch by frosting, if desired. Combine and beat at high speed until creamy: 1 8-ounce package cream cheese, ⅓ cup honey, and 1 tablespoon orange rind. Refrigerate cake if frosted.

Carob Snack Cake

This cake stores and travels well.

¾ cup whole-wheat flour
½ cup unbleached all-purpose flour
½ cup brown sugar
¼ cup arrowroot or cornstarch
1 teaspoon baking soda
½ cup maple syrup
¼ cup carob powder or cocoa
¾ cup black coffee
⅓ cup oil
1 tablespoon vinegar
1 teaspoon vanilla

Preheat oven to 350°. Mix dry ingredients in an ungreased 9-inch square baking pan. Make a well in the center; add remaining ingredients. Mix together with a fork until smooth. Bake 30–35 minutes. Cool in pan before sprinkling with confectioners sugar, if desired. Cut in squares to serve.

Apple Snack Cake

2 tablespoons butter or margarine
1 cup brown sugar, packed
1 egg
3 cups pared, diced apples
½ cup chopped nuts
1 teaspoon vanilla
1 cup unbleached flour
¼ teaspoon salt
¼ teaspoon cinnamon
1 teaspoon baking soda

Preheat oven to 350. Cream together butter, sugar, and egg. Stir in apples, nuts, and vanilla. Combine remaining ingredients and add to apple mixture; mix well. Turn into greased and floured 9 × 5 × 3-inch pan. Bake 50–60 minutes. Cool 15 minutes before removing from pan.

Whole Wheat Maple Cake

A very easy recipe that makes a nice breakfast "treat" as well.

1 cup maple syrup
½ cup vegetable oil or melted butter
1 teaspoon each: cloves, nutmeg, cinnamon, salt
1 cup seedless raisins
1 cup cold water
1 ¾ cups whole-wheat flour*
¼ cup cornstarch
1 teaspoon baking soda
½ cup chopped nuts

Place syrup, oil, spices, raisins, and water in saucepan. Bring to boil and boil for 4 minutes. Chill thoroughly in refrigerator.

Preheat oven to 350°. Sift together the whole-wheat flour, cornstarch, and baking soda three times. Add to the boiled mixture along with the nuts. Beat well. Pour into greased 9 × 5 × 3-inch pan. Bake 60 minutes. Cool in pan.

* 2 cups unbleached all-purpose flour may be substituted for the whole-wheat flour and cornstarch. Sift only once with the baking soda.

Spice Snack Cake

A really quick blender cake recipe.

> 1½ cups sifted unbleached flour
> 2 teaspoons baking powder
> ½ teaspoon salt
> ½ teaspoon each: cinnamon, cloves, nutmeg, allspice
> ⅓ cup shortening or vegetable oil
> ⅔ cup milk
> 1 large egg
> 1 cup light brown sugar, packed

Preheat oven to 350°. Sift together dry ingredients into bowl. Place remaining ingredients in blender in order listed; blend until smooth. Pour blended mixture gradually into sifted mixture, stirring lightly until just smooth. Pour into greased and floured 8-inch square pan. Bake 35 minutes. Cool in pan.

Plain Cake: Substitute 1 teaspoon vanilla for spices.

Banana Spice Cake: Substitute ¾ cup mashed banana and ¼ cup milk and ¼ teaspoon baking soda for the ⅔ cup milk. Add ⅓ cup chopped nuts and ⅓ cup chopped raisins.

Jam Cake

> ¾ cup soft margarine
> 3 eggs
> 1 cup brown sugar
> 1 cup jam (preferably red)
> 1 cup whole-wheat flour
> 1½ cups unbleached all-purpose flour
> 1 teaspoon baking soda
> ¾ cup yogurt
> ¼ cup brandy

Preheat oven to 350°. Cream margarine until fluffy. Blend in eggs, sugar, and jam; beat 2 minutes. Stir in flour and baking soda alternately with combined yogurt and brandy; stir until smooth. Spoon into a greased and floured 9 × 5 × 3-inch pan. Bake 50–60 minutes. Cool in pan; turn out onto wire rack to finish cooling.

Dandy Candy

Even younger members of the family can make these themselves.

¼ cup peanut butter
¼ cup buttermilk powder*
2 tablespoons chopped raisins
3-4 tablespoons maple syrup
Shredded coconut

Combine all ingredients, *except* coconut, until of kneadable consistency. Roll teaspoonfuls into balls; roll balls in shredded coconut. Makes about 16 candies.

Add crunch by rolling candies in nuts, sesame or sunflower seeds instead of coconut.

Add punch to dried dates or prunes by stuffing them with candy mixture.

* Dried skim milk powder may be substituted for all or part of the buttermilk powder but buttermilk powder makes a "sweeter" candy.

Sweet Sesame Treats

1 cup honey
1 cup peanut butter
1 cup cocoa or carob powder
1 cup sesame seeds
1 cup sunflower seeds
Grated or shredded coconut

Combine honey, peanut butter, cocoa, sesame seeds, and sunflower seeds in mixing bowl; mix with electric mixer until well mixed. Form into balls and roll in coconut. Freeze until firm.

Crunchy Fruit Munch

This favorite recipe is from the American Pop Corn Company.

3 quarts freshly popped Jolly Time Pop Corn
2 cups natural cereal with raisins
¾ cup dried apricots, chopped
¼ teaspoon salt
⅓ cup butter or margarine
¼ cup honey

Preheat oven to 300°. Combine first four ingredients in large baking pan. Set aside. In small saucepan, combine butter *or* margarine and honey. Cook over low heat until butter or margarine is melted. Pour over popcorn mixture, tossing lightly until well coated. Place in oven. Bake 30 minutes, stirring occasionally. Makes 3 quarts. Cool before storing in tightly covered container for up to two weeks.

Apple Spice Fruit Leather

1 pound apples, washed, peeled, and cored
¼ cup apple juice (about)
¼ teaspoon cinnamon
¼ teaspoon almond extract
1 cup ground or finely chopped nuts

Cut apples into chunks. Place in blender with as little apple juice as necessary to blend; blend to purée. Pour into bowl; stir in cinnamon and almond extract.

Line a cookie sheet with plastic wrap or spray with a non-stick vegetable spray. Spread purée evenly, leaving a 1-inch wide border all around. Sprinkle with nuts. Dry in oven at lowest possible temperature (under 200°) or over pilot light until no longer moist and sticky. Peel off plastic wrap; roll up. Slice at intervals and wrap in plastic wrap to store.

Mixed Fruit Leather

1 16-ounce can apricots, liquid included
1 pound pears, cored, peeled, and sliced
1 pound apples, cored, peeled, and sliced
1 tablespoon lemon juice
1 tablespoon honey

Place all ingredients in a blender; blend to purée. Follow directions for *Apple Spice Fruit Leather* above, using 2 or 3 lined cookie sheets.

Crunch and Munch Snax

1 cup almonds
1 cup peanuts
1 cup unsweetened coconut
1 cup cashews or *sunflower seeds*
2 tablespoons oil
1 cup dried apples, chopped
½ teaspoon cinnamon

Preheat oven to 300°. Mix all ingredients *except* apples and cinnamon. Spread on two greased cookie sheets and bake 20 minutes. Stir in apples and cinnamon. Cool completely before storing in covered container or packaging single servings in plastic sandwich bags.

Crunch Carob Candy

½ cup peanut or *almond butter*
½ cup sunflower seeds, ground
¼ cup sesame seeds, preferably toasted
½ cup minced dates
1 tablespoon carob powder
1 tablespoon honey or *date sugar*
2 tablespoons carob powder (additional) mixed with
*   3 tablespoons date sugar or grated coconut*

Mix first six ingredients until well blended. Form into small balls and roll in the carob and date sugar or coconut. Store in covered container or wrap in plastic wrap. Refrigerate. Makes 2 dozen.

Graham Cracker Candy Bars

10 (double) plain or cinnamon graham crackers (or enough to
*   line pan)*
1 cup margarine
1 cup maple syrup, honey, or brown sugar
1 cup chopped walnuts or *½ cup each coconut and chocolate*
*   chips*

Preheat oven to 350°. Line a 10 × 15 × 1-inch jellyroll pan with foil and grease well. Break crackers along perforations and arrange quartered crackers in pan. Mix remaining ingredients in a saucepan. Melt over low heat; then bring to a boil over medium heat. Continue cooking, stirring several times, for 2 minutes. Pour over crackers, spreading if needed to cover all crackers. Bake 10 minutes *only*. (Have faith; they will harden as they cool.) Cool before cutting into bars along lines formed by crackers.

Fancy Fig Candy

½ cup minced dried figs
½ cup minced dates
¼ cup tahini or nut butter
½ cup coconut, preferably unsweetened

Combine first three ingredients until well blended. Form into small balls. Roll in coconut. Store, covered, in refrigerator or cool place. Makes about 20.

Caramel Corn

4 quarts popped popcorn
1 cup peanuts
⅔ cup molasses
1⅓ cups maple syrup
1 tablespoon hot water
¼ teaspoon baking soda
2 teaspoons oil or margarine
½ teaspoon vinegar

Combine popcorn and peanuts in large bowl. Bring the molasses and maple syrup to a boil in large saucepan. Boil, stirring frequently, until temperature reaches 260° on candy thermometer (or forms a hard ball when tested in cold water). Stir baking soda into hot water and add to syrup along with oil or margarine and vinegar. Stir briskly for 1 minute longer. Pour over popcorn and peanuts; stirring to mix. Spread on greased cookie sheets to cool. Break apart when cool and store in covered containers or plastic bags.

9: *What's Good for Lunch?*

School lunches (served at school) are based on a formula that provides more than one-third of the Recommended Daily Allowance of nutrients. Each child gets two ounces of protein, at least three-fourths cup of fruit and vegetables (served as two or more items), a serving of bread and a half-pint of milk.

You can follow the same basic plan to provide nutritious brown bag lunches, using foods you know your family members will eat. Use this guide to plan luncheon menus that will follow the same guidelines that have been established for school lunch programs. Try to provide one-third of the recommended number of daily servings in each lunch.

THE MEAT AND MEAT ALTERNATES GROUP

Foods in this group include:
Meat
Poultry
Seafood
Eggs
Dry beans
Dry peas
Lentils
Nuts
Peanut butter

Recommended number of daily servings:
2 or more

Examples of one serving:
3 ounces lean cooked meat, poultry, or
    fish (without bone)
2 eggs
1 cup cooked dry beans, peas, or lentils
4 tablespoons peanut butter

THE MILK AND MILK PRODUCTS GROUP

Foods in this group include:
Milk: fluid, whole, dry
    evaporated
    skim or nonfat
    Buttermilk
    Yogurt
Cheese: Cottage cheese
    Cream cheese
    Cheddar-type
        cheeses
    natural cheeses
    process cheeses
Ice cream

Recommended number of daily servings:
    (in terms of 8-ounce cups of milk)
Children   3 cups or more
Teenagers   4 cups or more
Adults   2 cups or more
Pregnant women   3 cups or more
Nursing mothers   4 cups or more
Examples of one serving:
1 cup milk or plain yogurt *or* 1⅓ ounce
    Cheddar cheese
2 ounces process cheese
2 cups cottage cheese
4 tablespoons Parmesan cheese
1½ cups ice cream or ice milk

THE VEGETABLES AND FRUITS GROUP

Foods in this group include:
All vegetables and fruits, including the following good sources of vitamins A or C:
Apricots (A)
Broccoli (A, C)
Brussels sprouts (C)
Cantaloupe (A)
Carrots (A)
Dark, leafy greens (A)
Deep yellow vegetables (A)
Grapefruit (C)
Mango (A, C)
Oranges (C)
Peppers (C)
Pumpkin (A)
Spinach (A)
Strawberries (C)
Sweet potatoes (A)

Recommended number of daily servings:
4 or more, including:
1 serving of a good source of vitamin C
1 serving of a good source of vitamin A
and
2 or 3 servings any vegetable or fruit including potatoes and additional servings of those valuable for vitamin C and vitamin A

Examples of one serving:
½ cup cooked vegetable or fruit
1 cup cut-up raw vegetable or fruit
1 typical portion such as: 1 medium apple, banana, orange, or potato
½ medium grapefruit or cantaloupe
½ cup juice

THE BREADS AND CEREALS GROUP

Foods in this group include:
Whole grain or enriched breads
Cooked or ready-to-eat cereals
Bulgur
Cornmeal
Grits
Rice
Pasta
Baked Goods

Recommended number of daily servings:
4 or more

Examples of one serving:
1 slice bread
1 ounce ready-to-eat cereal
½–¾ cup cooked cereal, cornmeal, grits, or rice
½–¾ cup noodles, macaroni, spaghetti or other pasta

EATING FOR BETTER HEALTH SUBSTITUTIONS

Making relatively small changes in the foods you eat or prepare for your family can improve the nutritional quality and variety of your diet. The suggestions presented here are based on the Dietary Guidelines published jointly by the U.S. Departments of Agriculture and Health and Human Resources.

Instead of this ingredient:	Use this ingredient:
Beef, regular ground (20% fat)	Lean ground beef (11% fat)
Beef bouillon, canned or cubes	Homemade, defatted beef broth
Bread crumbs for topping	Bread crumbs + wheat germ
Butter, 1 cup	= ⅔ cup vegetable oil
Catsup	Reduced sodium recipe on page 127
Chocolate, 1 ounce	= ¼ cup carob or cocoa + 1 teaspoon oil
Cottage cheese	Tofu (soy bean curd)
Cream, light	Undiluted evaporated milk
Cream, sour, 1 cup	= ½ cup yogurt + ½ cup cottage cheese + 2 teaspoons lemon juice
Cream cheese, regular	Light cream cheese or Yogurt Cheese, page 52
Creamer, non-dairy	Undiluted evaporated skim milk
Eggs, whole, 2	= 1 whole egg + 2 egg whites + 1 teaspoon oil
Flour, white, 1 cup	= ⅞ cup whole-wheat flour
Fruit, canned sweetened	Juice pack fruit
Gelatin dessert, fruit flavored	Plain gelatin + fruit juice
Half-and-half	Undiluted evaporated skim milk
Milk, whole	Low fat milk; apple juice, water, vegetable broth, or soy milk also make good substitutes for cooking and baking
Peanut butter, homogenized	Natural—not hydrogenated—peanut butter
Rice, white or instant	Brown rice
Tuna, packed in oil	Water pack tuna
Water	Liquid from cooking vegetables or draining unsweetened fruit
Sherry, cooking	Dry white wine
Yogurt, fruit flavored	Plain yogurt + fresh fruit
Tomatoes, canned	Tomato paste or purée, canned

PACK SOME PUNCH IN YOUR LUNCH

Add variety to lunches by changing the texture and flavor of your favorite recipes. Chef's Salad becomes Antipasto Salad with a change of meats and the addition of chick peas—or go Polynesian by substituting chicken for the meat and cheese and adding pineapple in place of the usual tomato. Give spaghetti a fiery Mexican flair by substituting chili powder and cayenne—or go Indonesian with a little curry in your pilaf.

Foods That Go "Crunch" When You Munch:

alfalfa sprouts
bacon (freeze crumbled bits for adding to egg or chicken salad)
chick peas (garbanzos)
cornmeal (sprinkle on breads and crackers before baking
croutons (soups, salads, casseroles)
fruit, raw: crisp apples, grapes, pears, pineapple
granola
mung bean sprouts
nuts
oats (for topping baked goods)
peanuts
sesame seeds (sprinkle on bread, cakes, rolls before baking)
sunflower seeds (add to salads, sprinkle on baked goods)
vegetables, raw: asparagus tips, crisp broccoli, carrots, cauliflower, celery, scallions
water chestnuts
wheat germ (sprinkle on casseroles before baking, add to breads)

Foods That Add Punch To Your Lunch:

cayenne pepper
curry (nice change in mayonnaise)
horseradish (try in dips; adds zest to meatloaf)
hot pepper sauce (adds snap to eggs)
lemon juice or rind
mustard (zaps up your mayonnaise)
olives
pickles (chopped in sandwich fillings)
pickling liquid (use leftovers for marinating or vinaigrette)
pimientos (great color!)
radish seed sprouts
watercress (a peppery flavor for salad)

Pack a Surprise:

A newspaper or magazine clipping you think your spouse would enjoy.
A greeting card when it's a special day.
An invitation to a special after school snack, trip to the zoo, candlelight dinner, movie that night.
An inexpensive game, puzzle, toy, comic book—especially if it's a rainy day and you know outside activities will be curtailed.
A special candy treat from Chapter 8.
For yourself, a good book you've been wanting to read.
A book of jokes or cartoons you've clipped to share with co-workers.

10: Menus for Anybody...
Anytime...Anywhere

*see Index for recipes

TAKE-OUT BREAKFASTS

Breakfast Quiche-to-Go*
Fruit and Nut Turnover*
Hot cocoa or carob drink

Morning Fruit Cup*
Oatmeal Muffin*   Beverage

Morning Glory*
Bacony Breakfast Cookies*

Apple Juice
Breakfast Bulgur*
Blueberry Muffin*   Milk

Golden Eggnog*
Winter Fruit and Nut Turnovers*
Beverage

Orange Juice
Brown Rice Pudding* with milk
Beverage

Grapefruit Juice
Appealing Apricot Bread*
with cream cheese
Beverage

Orange Juice
All-in-One Micro Breakfast*
Beverage

Tangerine
Yogurt sprinkled with cinnamon
Apple Butter Muffin*   Beverage

Nut Butter Spread* in pita bread
Orange or apple   Beverage

KID STUFF

BLT Rice*
Sunshine Salad*
Peanut Butter Apple Cookies*
Milk

Chilly Tomato Soup*
Vegetable Wheat Crackers*
Celery stuffed with cheese
Crunchy Fruit Munch*   Juice

Devilish Chicken Fingers*
Tabbouleh* or New Potato Salad*
Dill pickle slices*
Graham Cracker*   Pear   Milk

Cream cheese or cottage cheese
on Sweet 'n' Snappy Pear Bread*
Raw vegetable sticks
Carob Chip Cookie*   Apple Juice

Golden Garbanzo Loaf* in pita
Quick Coleslaw*
Pineapple Bars*   Milk

Hearty Wintertime Spaghetti*
Cheese Wedges   Vegetable sticks
Fantastic Fig Bars*   Juice

Peanut butter and raisin sandwich
Ruby applesauce*
Pudding or frozen fruit yogurt
Milk or Juice

Egg and Almond filling*
on Burger Buns*
Sweet Pickles*   Carrot sticks
Overnight Bread Pudding*   Juice

EVERYBODY'S FAVORITES

Barely Beef Chili*
Cornbread*
Raw Vegetable Sticks
Jim Jams*   Apple   Milk

Tuna salad on Rolled Rye Bread*
Zucchini and carrot sticks
Orange Apple Nut Bar*   Milk

Crunchy Summertime Spaghetti*
Tossed Green Salad
with Basic Salad Dressing*
Carob Snack Cake*   Beverage

Chicken Loaf* on rye bread
Cranberry Apple Waldorf Mold*
Oat Crunchies*   Milk

Hearty Wintertime Spaghetti*
Quick Bread Sticks*
Raw vegetable sticks
Fruit cocktail   Milk

Turkey Meatballs* in pita bread
Every-ready Coleslaw*
Fruit   Beverage

Mandarin Special Salad*
with Almond Dressing*
Orange Muffins*
Yogurt with fresh fruit   Beverage

Sliced chicken on Onion Roll*
Bean Salad*   or vegetable sticks
Pumpkin Cookie*   Pear   Milk

Tabbouleh* with tuna added
Vegetable sticks
Jelly Bars*   Milk or beverage

Creamy Molded Chicken Salad*
Cranberry Banana Bread*
Sweet Sesame Treats*   Beverage

DIET DELIGHTS

Cold poached chicken
Tossed green salad
with Low Calorie Dressing*
Low-fat yogurt with fresh fruit

Great Grape Take-a-Shake*
Melba toast   Peach or orange

Ham and Cheese Roll-ups*
Celery and pepper sticks
Nutty Rye Crackers*
Peach   Low calorie beverage

Ham or chicken sticks
Yogurt Cheese*
on Vegetable Wheat Thins*
Celery and carrot sticks
Fresh strawberries or peach   Tea

Quick Clam Chowder*
Cheese wedges   Melba toast
Low-fat yogurt with fruit   Tea

Water packed tuna
on Tossed Green Salad
Carrot and zucchini sticks
Cherry tomatoes
Melba toast or Wheat Thins*
Grapefruit   Tea

Lime Chicken*
Springtime Vegetable Mold*
Melba Toast
Fruit   Tea

Hi-Pro Take-a-Shake*
Apple Butter Muffin*
Beverage

Very Vegetable Soup*
Vegetable Wheat Thins*
Fresh fruit or yogurt
Beverage

Index

Other Books from Betterway Publications

HOMEMAKING GUIDES & HANDBOOKS

OCCUPATION: HOMEMAKER by Sharron K. Lamb. A tribute to the original "working woman." Covers the rewards and challenges of her life today and the opportunities available after the child-raising years in words that are sometimes impassioned, sometimes humorous—but never dull. *Paperback, illustrated, 140 pages, $5.95.*

Jackie's HOME REPAIR & MAINTENANCE CHARTS by Richard G. Mills, edited by Jacqueline Hostage. A basic guide to home upkeep. All routine maintenance and repair chores covered in easy to follow, step-by-step guides; what tools to use, what to do, when and how to do it. The unhandy-person's best friend. *Paperback, illustrated, 128 pages, comb-bound, $5.95.*

Jackie's INDOOR/OUTDOOR GARDENING CHARTS by Jacqueline Hostage. A comprehensive collection of charts, pointers, step-by-step guides, and grow-how notes that cover all aspects of gardening—from planning and planting to maintenance. *Paperback, illustrated, 128 pages, comb-bound, $5.95.*

Jackie's BOOK OF HOUSEHOLD CHARTS by Jacqueline Hostage. The ultimate homemaker's helper, with house and garden tips, information on family nutrition, food storage and preparation, keeping family records, coping with inflation, much more. *Paperback, illustrated, 112 pages, comb-bound, $5.95.*

BOOKS FOR COOKS

DOES YOUR LUNCH PACK PUNCH? by Robin Toth and Jacqueline Hostage. A cookbook for the crunch & munch bunch that offers more than 200 super recipes for eating at home or brown bagging. Includes a special section on the newest packaging products available to lunch toters. *Paperback, photographs, 160 pages, $6.95.*

Jackie's KITCHEN CHARTS by Jacqueline Hostage. A practical guide to kitchen management with charts covering food preparation, storage, and preservation; buying and cooking guides; inventory charts; kitchen formulas; much more. *Paperback, illustrated, 128 pages, comb-bound, $5.95.*

COOKING FOR LOVE...AND MONEY by Evelyn Kirk Kennedy. Written by a woman who was a nationally-syndicated food columnist for years, this book tells readers how to earn money and prizes by entering and winning contests, selling recipes, holding cooking classes, more. *Hardcover— $10.95, paperback—176 pages, $6.95.*

PERSONAL SAFETY

HOW TO AVOID TRAFFIC TICKETS by Edward R. Smith. Written by a veteran police officer. Covers every issue of importance to both new and seasoned drivers and takes the mystery out of all the laws and regulations. Inside advice on how to behave if stopped by a police officer. *Illustrated paperback, 80 pages, $3.95.*

FAMILY HEALTH & NUTRITION

AM I STILL VISIBLE?—A Woman's Triumph Over Anorexia Nervosa by Sandra H. Heater. An important book for those who are—or may become —victims of anorexia nervosa; their family and friends; and the professionals who treat this insidious illness. A powerful autobiography with an excellent research and treatment section. *Hardcover—$10.95, paperback— 140 pages, $6.95.*

LIVING...WITHOUT MILK by Jacqueline Hostage. A reference source, nutritional guide, and alternative cookbook for individuals who are lactose intolerant or allergic to dairy products. Approved by medical and nutrition authorities. *Hardcover—$7.95, paperback—140 pages, $3.95.*

Jackie's DIET & NUTRITION CHARTS by Jacqueline Hostage. A good health maintenance and weight control program for thinking adults. Includes NUTRI-DIET®, a simple system for safe, quick weight loss. *Paperback, illustrated, 128 pages, comb-bound, $5.95.*

SMALL & HOME BUSINESS GUIDES

SMALL BUSINESSES THAT GROW AND GROW AND GROW by Patricia A. Woy. An information-packed small business guide and handbook. Detailed descriptions of small business opportunities for everyone from shoestring entrepreneurs (less than $100) to those with more than $10,000 to invest. *Paperback, 208 pages, $7.95.*

THE BEST OF BOTH WORLDS—A Guide To Home-Based Careers by Joan Wester Anderson. Written especially for the woman who wants to fulfill herself without sacrificing the values of a strong family life. Packed with practical advice and scores of ideas. *Hardcover—$10.95, paperback— 188 pages, $6.95.*

PARENTING

TEEN IS A FOUR-LETTER WORD—A Survival Kit For Parents by Joan Wester Anderson. Focuses with insight, empathy, and humor on all the important teen stages. Offers solid counsel on both traditional problems (dating, school hours, etc.) and the more contemporary problems of sexual activity, alcohol use, and drug abuse. *Paperback, 140 pages, $5.95.*

BOOKS FOR CREATIVE YOUNG PEOPLE

MY MOST MARVELOUS MEMORY BOOK—A Special Diary For Young People by Judith King. A beautifully-produced book for youngsters in the 10 to 14 age group. Encourages them to record all their important growing-up memories and dreams. A lovely gift for a favorite daughter, granddaughter, niece, or family friend. *Comb-bound paperback, 7×10, 64 pages, $6.95.*

NATURALLY IT'S GOOD...I cooked it myself! by Robin Toth. This cookbook and nutritional guide for kids in the 10 to 14 age group makes cooking and eating sensibly fun. 140 delicious recipes help kids learn basic cooking skills while they learn about good nutrition. *Hardcover, 176 pages, $9.95.*

SEWING & CRAFTS

THE SEW & SAVE SOURCE BOOK—Your Guide To Supplies For Creative Sewing by Margaret A. Boyd. An all-inclusive directory of more than 1500 mail-order suppliers for at-home sewing needs. Everything from supplies, kits, and patterns to tools, equipment, and services. Scores of available books, trade publications, magazines, and educational services. *Paperback, photographs, illustrated, 8½ × 11, 208 pages, $9.95.*

FAMILY FUN

THE WIT & WISDOM OF ANON.—Humor by Marjorie C. Mahoney. A collection of smile-makers, rib-ticklers, and belly-laughers from the pen of Anonymous. Quips, anecdotes, definitions, and limericks you can use as your own. *Hardcover, 96 pages, $5.95.*

THE GREATEST GIFT GUIDE EVER by Judith King. A book that helps bring thoughtfulness and originality to the gift-giving process. Innovative and complete, with more than 3200 gift ideas arranged into 81 categories. *Paperback, 190 pages, $5.95.*

MY PERSONAL GIFT PROFILES by Judith King. A desk-quality companion booklet to THE GREATEST GIFT GUIDE EVER. Helps plan and record the perfect gifts you give family and friends. *Paperback, 48 pages, $2.95.*

UNPUZZLING YOUR PAST—A Basic Guide To Genealogy by Emily Anne Croom. A complete how-to guide and handybook for the beginning genealogist. Shows readers how to trace their roots by combining the use of living sources with research into public records. Includes more than twenty reproducible forms. *Paperback, illustrated, 128 pages, 8½ × 11, $7.95.*